COVID-19: Illness & Illumination

A Hypnotic Exploration

by

Lincoln Stoller, PhD, CHt

MindStrengthBalance.com

Also by Lincoln Stoller, published by MindStrengthBalance.com:

~

The Learning Project: Rites of Passage,

Becoming Lucid: Self-Awareness in Sleeping & Waking Life,

The Path To Sleep: Exercises for an Ancient Skill.

COVID-19
ILLNESS & ILLUMINATION

a hypnotic exploration

Lincoln Stoller, PhD, CHt

First Edition.
Published 2020 by Mind Strength Balance
Victoria, British Columbia, Canada
https://www.mindstrengthbalance.com

Stoller, Lincoln, 1956- author.
covid-19 : illness and illumination / Lincoln Stoller.
ISBN 978-1-9992538-8-2 (mobi) | ISBN 978-1-9992538-7-5 (epub)
ISBN 978-1-9992538-5-1 (paper) | ISBN 978-1-9992538-6-8 (hard cover)
ISBN 978-1-9992538-9-9 (audio)

Subjects: LCSH: Hypnotism—Therapeutic use. | Suggestive therapeutics. | Disease management. | Epidemics. | Ecological disasters.

Cover Art, paintings by:
Alexander von Humboldt
Hans Grabner
Back Cover Art by:
Charles Smith

Praise for COVID-19: Illness and Illumination

Finally, a thoughtful approach to the COVID-19 pandemic! Dr. Stoller seamlessly combines the ineluctable substance of our natural milieu with the hard facts that now confront us, in a manner reminiscent of George Engel's biopsychosocial model of medicine. The additional resource of medical hypnotherapy, added in sensible measures to reduce stress and improve natural immunity, makes for a compelling argument, intended to aid in earlier diagnosis and more effective treatment. Pandemics are not new, and we again realize the frailty of our human condition. Dr. Stoller has provided needed aids in combating this crisis, and those to come.

— **George Plotkin**, PhD, MD, Medical Director, UT Northeast Neurological Institute, and Associate Professor, Department of Internal Medicine, University of Texas, Tyler

~

It is vital that this much-needed information reaches the public. *COVID-19: Illness & Illumination* is a well-researched and important contribution at this time. What makes this book even more special is that the author combines his research with his knowledge and experience as a professional hypnotherapist. His "mind in matter" approach is based on the fact that the mind can influence the body. Dr. Stoller explains this process with exercises to benefit the readers.

— **Roy Hunter**, CHt, hypnotherapist, trainer, author of eight books on hypnosis

~

In *COVID-19: Illness & Illumination* he has created a map of learning, growth, and development. Dr. Lincoln Stoller is a provocative thinker with an easy to follow way of speaking and writing about complex topics and a calming effect. Dr. Stoller applies all his tools to address the changes, opportunities, and challenges for human health in the context of COVID-19. He provides a reassuring approach to well being in this time of powerful transformation.

— **Monica Geers Dahl**, EdD, CHt, IMDHA Life Diplomat in Hypnotherapy

Table of Contents

Acknowledgments

Clearly, the SARS family of viruses deserves the lion's share of the credit and the blame. If there is a silver lining to be found, it resides in the virus's forcing us toward new thought, greater collaboration, and better understanding.

Unfortunately, there are clouds on the horizon. In an increasingly strained and competitive world, it is escaping no one that a pandemic doesn't affect everyone equally. There are big losers and there might be big winners.

If an epidemic can be harnessed, then it is a near perfect weapon: cheap, fast, blameless, indefatigable, and almost unstoppable—at least for those without an antidote. The greatest risk lies in a pathogen's unpredictable power and its ability to mutate out of control. And while biological warfare is banned by treaty, the selective release of natural forces is not.

Seeing how governments behave, I'm sure they're thinking about it. To harness a virus is like hitting the jackpot: it can destroy competing economies leaving alliances and resources intact. You don't even have to declare war, you just win!

Modern civilization, with its codependent economies, has outgrown territorial wars out of necessity, but not out of choice. Future wars will be fought over energy, data, and resources. Mechanical armies are increasingly obsolete; the future is digital and ecological.

Humanity will and has done more damage to itself than any ecological force. Time after time, the ecology has shown us how to balance growth with stability, but we have not gotten the memo. COVID-19 is that memo writ large and nailed to every door. It would be nice if this was the pandemic to end all pandemics. If that came to pass, we might give SARS-CoV-2 more credit than blame.

Prologue

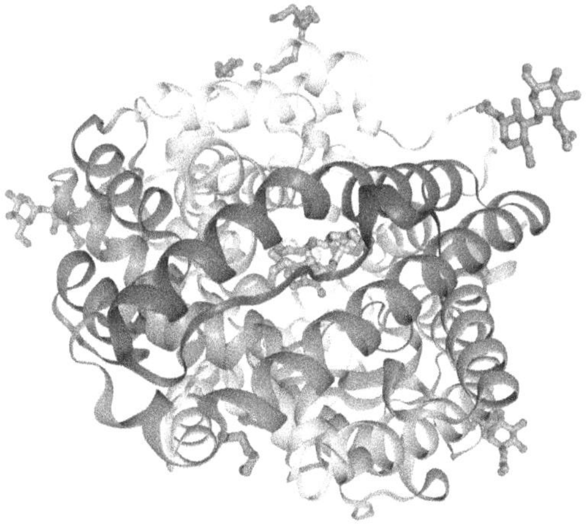

The ACE2 Protein structure to which SARS-CoV-2 bonds in order to enter a cell.

"Each essay was designed to be complete in itself; and one and the same tendency pervades the whole…"
— **Alexander von Humboldt** (Humboldt 1850, p.ix)

These chronicles mix physics, medicine, hypnotherapy, technology, culture, learning, politics, and the news surrounding the Coronavirus from March through June of 2020. This is the first phase of the pandemic, before the expected second infection, and before any vaccine.

This mixing of perspectives is unusual. Few authors have the background to support it. Fewer recognize that integrating many perspectives is necessary to understand what has and is continuing to happen. The virus is not one thing having many impacts; it is many things happening with the virus at the center.

To some extent, this is true of any historical event. Human events and nature, in general, do not follow a storyline. It is more accurate—in fact, it is essential in this case—to include the full extent of the disorder when trying to understand the situation. The pandemic has many aspects.

The situation cannot be understood without considering the chaotic forces and policies that formed it. There is no "one story;" no one authoritative point of view; no single, resolving explanation. Any such orderly presentation of events—and there will be many as various pundits, experts, and spokespeople present their cases—is one slice through a multi-dimensional event.

These chapters are chronological, written weekly in the order in which they occurred. A summary relationship of all the chapters is given in chapter one. Putting events in order does not mean the events are orderly, even though one wants to discern order as events unfold.

Much of what becomes evident has been brewing for years—maybe centuries—hidden in policies, bureaucracies, attitudes, economies, cultures, ecological injury, and other dynamics whose combustible elements were either segregated, inactive, unrecognized or mutating toward this trigger point.

My work focuses on complex systems; systems that involve multiple disciplines, skills, attitudes, people, backgrounds, and cultures. I have practiced in many fields, from science to sociology, technology to art, theory and experiment. I have worked with youth and elders from various cultures around the world. I continue to bring these disciplines together in my work as an explorer, entrepreneur, author, therapist, consultant, neuroscientist, and physicist.

I am concerned with the quality of information. A recent analysis using an information quality tool called DISCERN, applied to information on COVID-19 available through YouTube videos, has shown this information to be poor (Szmuda, 2020). The DISCERN tool rates information on the basis of its aims, clarity, relevance, balance, support, and risk/benefit discussion. I hope this book rates highly on these criteria.

Lincoln Stoller, 2020

www.mindstrengthbalance.com and www.mindstrengthbooks.com.

Follow @LincolnStoller and #IllnessAndIllumination

Note to the Reader

Each chapter in this book ends with a hypnotic session presenting the material in a manner that engages your emotions and detaches you from your senses. However, if you are reading this, then you may not benefit from these sessions since the act of reading contains you within a nonemotional, verbal state of mind. To gain the most benefit from these sessions, they should be read to you.

To make this possible for readers of the text, at the start of each session, I have included a link to folder on the internet that contains MP3 sound files which you can download. In this folder there is a sound file for each hypnotic session, and you may listen to these files at your convenience. They may put you to sleep but, as long as it is a light sleep, you will hear and appreciate them.

The URL for this folder is:

https://www.mindstrengthbalance.com/covid19-illness-illumination/

— CAUTION —

Do not listen to these audio files while driving a car, operating machinery, or doing anything that requires your attention!

I – COVID-19 Chronicles

More than a human infection: canary in a coal mine.

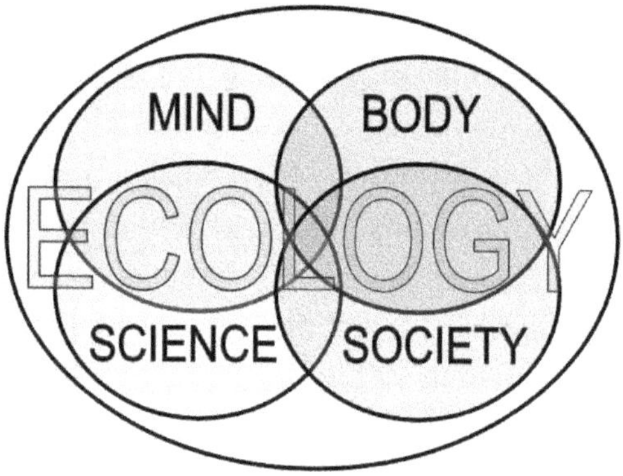

"Human health is the great global connector."
— **Kathleen Sebelius**, former US Secretary of Health and Human Services

Interconnections

Things that do not connect to us do not exist for us, which means we only see what relates to us. That doesn't mean everything that's connected to us is connected to everything else. Rather, it's a network, and networks have many structures.

We are connected to rocks, we use them for foundations. But from a rock's point of view, we play no role in their geology. If I hit you with a rock it's bad news for you, but hitting a rock with you means nothing to a rock. The nature of the connection makes all the difference.

For our simple minds, things are connected in either one or both directions. That is, the connection either goes one way or both ways. We think of one-way connections as inert because the object in a one-way connection is unresponsive: nothing comes back. That describes our connection to rocks.

A two-way connection creates a dialog and the connection becomes part of a complex or a system. There is feedback; there are consequences. People form systems with other people. People form connections with elements in their ecology.

I look for two-way connections. Two-way connections create things that are greater than one-way, cause and effect. New identities arise from systems that foster the creation of new things. If there is a current, growth, and resonance, then these new things can appear life-like. Ecology arises from multiple two-way connections and it is a life-like thing. Ecology is a living thing even though it doesn't have a membrane around it. This is how we're looking at the virus: as a component of an ecological system.

Time

From our preconceived view of the world, we give time a special role. Because of this prejudice, we overlook similarities between time and space. Because we live in a time-trending universe—one in which we're all moving together through time and not one in which we're all moving together through space—we don't recognize as constant things that change in time. In spite of this, there are many similarities between structures that vary over time and structures that vary over space.

For example—as was recently described in the scientific literature—there are time crystals. These are things whose structures manifest stable, regular, and repeating patterns through time. There are many complex systems that, under the right conditions, fall into repeating patterns: ecologies, weather patterns, markets, people, and civilizations. These are some examples of the many things that our limited concept of time structures has prevented us from understanding.

We recognize things as separate when they persist separately without support. We identify a boundary as the container of a thing. We accept a thing as having some unique identity if it is constant along its boundary in spite of what may be changing inside its boundary.

We create boundaries around things so we can say they're separate. Then, we give them an identity. When that boundary fails—and that boundary may be a skin or another person's role in our lives—we see this as a kind of death. Such as the loss of a relationship with another, or outgrowing a part of ourselves.

We don't call it death when all of our cells are replaced within a month—

which they are—because our presentation to others and our sense of self remains the same. But if the presentation ends, then we recognize that something has ended and we call it "death." It's not our cessation of life that we recognize as death, it's our cessation of person-hood. The criteria of death are actually difficult to define and are rather arbitrary.

When it comes to looking at systems, we need to take a wider view. Systems are not just the things we see and recognize, they are also things that contain us and exist within us.

The COVID-19 pandemic is a system, it's a whole container of relationships. And this is not only because it has a cause and an effect, but also because it arises from previously disconnected elements and creates new relationships. These new systems—new ways of working, traveling, governing, considering, and forming conclusions—"crystallize" out of the cauldron of preceding affairs. Many of these systems will persist without the virus; they will not simply disappear when the virus disappears.

The structure that COVID-19 creates is not just an infection. It is that, but it also makes changes to the environment. The story of the virus's emergence—all the stories of the virus's emergence—are part of the pandemic's structure.

The final story that endures into the future will be labeled "history," but any one history is an illusion. There are other stories which may or may not be remembered: Latin, Anglo, and Afro; the rich and the poor, the urban and the rural, the uninfected, the survivor, and the casualty. The pandemic has triggered an avalanche of stories: economic, political, international, racial, and authoritarian. Which is the "real" story? Who will decide what we choose to forget?

The manner in which the disease unfolds is just as much a part of its structure as scientific facts, historical truths, or media hype. I have written this book to trace the structure that emerges following the path of a therapist-scientist-survivor-critic. The chronicle uses these four lenses. What comes into focus is not telescopic, but kaleidoscopic.

Truth

There is no more truth to any one history of COVID-19 than there is to social revolution, racial injustice, or the medical establishment. The virus provides a convenient hook on which to hang everything. Everything is the virus's fault and no one cares what the virus "thinks." We can reinvent the virus entirely.

But the virus does have a point of view. What it "thinks" is what it evolves to do, which is a function of the larger ecology we have created for it. From its point of view, none of our opinions have merit. The virus simply exploits a fertile niche until that resource becomes limited. From the virus's point of view, humanity is no different from a petri dish. We would be wise to recognize that in some situations, we are merely a resource to be mined, like oil.

This book looks at the virus like a time crystal: something precipitated into existence by an abrupt transition. It grew like a snowflake to encompass the earth. It will consolidate like a glacier and, eventually, move or melt and run into the sea. The sea, in this case, will be the collective pool of genetic material that the virus shares with us and the microbes within us.

This book is also a crystal. It starts at the time of the virus's emergence in North America's public awareness—which is coincident with my acquiring it. With each chapter, the contagion spreads through the world as it spreads through me. My case was mild, but it was significant. Because I am sensitive—and becoming sensitive is the theme of this book—I trace aspects of the disease that have only been described by people who've experienced different symptoms.

I experienced every symptom of the disease except the worst ones: I did not have lung symptoms, and I did not have organ failure. I have experienced—and in some cases continue to experience—upper respiratory, circulatory, neural, gastrointestinal, and epidermal symptoms. The neural symptoms include a continued soreness in the tissue of one foot, anxiety, and mood instability. The gastrointestinal symptoms manifest as a weakness in digestion, a sensitivity to processed foods, an adverse reaction to sugar, and a hunger for protein. The circulatory include general itching and occasional redness of my toes. I had—and still have—post-viral fatigue symptoms, which are only starting to be discussed, and which are not understood.

Reason

Today's culture increasingly rejects objectivity and, some would say, reason. The rejection of objectivity has been long in coming. On the other hand, reason is not what's being rejected, but rather deduction. That is because deduction requires facts, and when the facts are absent or corrupted, reason is reduced to authority. It's reduced to who has the authority to define the facts. Today's culture is rejecting authority.

The alternative to this kind of thinking—that which is seen as hostage to authority, which is to say deductive thinking—is inductive thinking. Support for inductive thinking is rising. The increasingly repressed culture—rich and poor—is being denied the power to define its world. And whether the leadership is benevolent, malevolent, patriarchal or matriarchal, if the situation forbids the chaos of growth, then it is repressive and will be resented.

In this situation, most people are being forced to accept the reasoning of a few. In particular, they're being forced to accept what authorities present as science. What's being presented is not science, because science is always skeptical, but people are miseducated to think that science means certainty. This misrepresentation is done intentionally to reduce chaos and improve political control.

This parallels the way parents defeat their children by using reason and authority. This abusive modeling denies a child's intuition and prevents learning. Abusive reason is just as much a failure in politics as it is in parenting. In both cases, you pay for it with chaos.

Inductive thinking is conjectural. It allows much wider conclusions and—while it is less accurate than deduction based on facts—its scope is more inclusive. In times of change, uncertainty, and multiplicity, the "real facts" are unknown or nonexistent. In these times, induction is more useful. Induction opens the paths of suspicion, whimsy, and creativity which deduction forbids until evidence allows.

We are exploring the mind's connection to the body where the nature of objectivity and subjectivity is ambiguous: you are what your mind sees of yourself, but there is more to you of which you are unaware. When we focus on ourselves, our distinctions between using objectivity and subjectivity—limiting ourselves to being reasonable—go out the window. If you want to find, become, or accept greater power, then you must recognize there is more to you than what you are aware of.

Disease

Everything is born from something; birthing something new requires the release of something old. In personal growth, there is always some part of you that you cannot bring along. In some cases this applies to healing; it certainly applies to psychosomatic issues. Psychosomatic healing involves a release.

All illness has a psychological aspect either in its inception, progression, or recovery. Finding health means losing illness; finding strength means losing weakness. We attach meaning to all our experiences, and we attach some part of ourselves to our illness and our weakness.

In some cases, our sense of vulnerability may precede our illness, in other cases, it may follow. It need not be causal at first—vulnerability leading to illness—but it can become causal once you have established the connection. You can use the connections you create in your mind to affect changes in your physical outcome.

You and your illness are not so unique. Your illness represents a vulnerability of our species. It's an experience we share as a culture. You can see this as simply the manner in which we have all been trained to deal with the experience. How we react to illness, whom we seek help from, and what support we expect.

There is a personal, learned aspect of our immunity. Our immune system does not operate entirely on its own, it learns at all levels: chemically, genetically, epigenetically, subconsciously, and consciously. And since some of this is taught to us, our immune system's learning also occurs socially.

This book approaches many aspects, but it does not consolidate them. Instead, it leaves separate threads because there is not one, objective story. Each of us will take these threads and weave a tapestry specific to ourselves—our own tartan of truth. This is how we take ownership: by creation, not by authority.

There is duplication in these chapters: points about diet, chemistry, microbes, information, and medicine. But the book's main purpose is not as a summary, but a resource, something to be used by those at risk of infection.

Individuals & Institutions

I consider many systems, from bio-molecules to species ecology, but there are two major systems I overlook. The first is how people understand things. The virus presents a learning opportunity and it reveals which people have successful learning skills, and which do not.

I am offering you a new perspective and a different experience. I'm assuming you'll understand it, but it won't make sense to everyone. Many of us have been taught to think linearly, either to follow authority or to limit ourselves to what has already been taught to us. To see things from a new perspective you'll need to open your mind.

The content in the first part of each chapter—the text—takes a rational approach, but the hypnotic journeys in the second part of each chapter do not. Every hypnotic induction starts by asking you to drop your reasoning mind, and this is too much for some people. Those people have bigger problems than being unable to follow this book: they also can't follow their intuition. Intuition exists in an emotional realm in which single conclusions don't exist.

The second issue I've overlooked is global politics. While SARS-CoV-2 is a virus, the situation it has created goes beyond an individual to a global illness.

This is not an infection, but it is an illness. It is our global geo-political dysfunction. I do not explore this; I can't, it's too large. But you will not understand what's happening at any human level—that is, outside of the molecular—without some understanding of the geo-politics.

There are hints that something is wrong in the suspiciously misguided or ineffective government responses. These are largely written off to ignorance, but they are not ignorant, they are all part of some strategy. It may not be the right strategy, and it may not be a strategy that's healthy for most people, in the short-term, or for you, but none of the institutional responses are baseless.

Few of the institutional responses are what they appear to be. Institutions primarily serve themselves and in chaotic times many of these institutions find themselves in conflict with each other. In the conflagration of COVID-19, many institutions are unsure of how to accomplish their own long-term goals. The layers of misrepresentation and disinformation may never be fully unraveled.

In the US, we are witnessing conflicts between the Executive and Legislative branches of government that began with the surprise election of Donald Trump as US President in 2016, a man whose only previous experience was as a financial dictator and TV game-show host. These conflicts have expanded to conflicts between federal, state, and municipal governments, and between military, social, and private sector services.

From roots of populism, poverty, racism, globalism, militarism, corporatism, and xenophobia—trends that have been growing in all the superpowers of the world and their satellites—we are now seeing toxic blooms in each cultural sphere. There are both accusations in the press and rioting in the streets.

The prevailing institutional conflict should not come as any surprise: it is the fight for global dominance. This is waged on two fronts: the control of money and the control of data. The player who controls the world's money controls the power. The player who controls the data controls the decisions.

We do not yet have global control of data. Each country is rushing to establish data hegemony within its boundaries and extend that control as far as possible. The reason the tech sector has become financially dominant is not just because they're selling smartphones, it's because they are selling the control of data and people as resources, and their major clients are governments.

Beneath product marketing are currents of collaboration, confederation, subterfuge, intelligence, espionage, security, and sabotage. This is what fuels conspiracy theories, and they're not false; they're just woefully inadequate.

We do have a global money system, but it's not stable. The fight for a dominant global currency, having been waged for decades out of the public eye—centuries, really: why do you think the Spanish wanted Montezuma's gold?—is now coming to a head in the conflict between the US dollar and the Chinese renminbi.

It doesn't really matter what currency is used, the issue is who controls it. This is the real reason that government responses to the pandemic have focused on securing their financial systems and extending their financial reach, not on the health of their citizenry.

Only one-tenth of the US government's financial response to the pandemic has addressed personal health; nine-tenths has gone to support corporate health. In the process, massive shifts of power—which were already underway—are centralizing institutional control of assets and data in all the superpowers. This is a continuation of war by other means.

Ecology

This book is about ecology and each of its chapters is a segment of this ecology. The pandemic can only be understood by bringing together its many pieces. Pieces that differ in size, affect various populations, and will persist over various scales of time.

Chapter one, this chapter **COIVD-19 Chronicles**, clarifies the connection between and the definition of things that concern us.

Chapter two, **Hypnosis For The New Flu**, takes things at face value. We look at things as they appear to be. COVID-19 appears to be a disease. It affects a person's breathing. There are no drugs to defeat it. It's spreading. Everyone is susceptible to it.

Chapter three, **The Lymphatic System**, steps away from the medical system to reflect on our body's natural response. This is compared with national and international responses, still at a face value level. I work to convince you of the third way: the way of your body.

Chapter four, **Become An Activist**, begins to show agitation as institutions bungle their efforts at advancing public health, and obvious, necessary actions are not taken. I admonish readers to become their own advocates and find their own information.

In chapter five, **Hypnosis for Your Lungs**, the discrepancy between individual needs and institutional initiatives is becoming clearer. Attention shifts as international news focuses on accusations and recrimination. The medical system struggles to cope as governments fail to supplement resources. Doctors trained to follow algorithms have none.

Chapter six, **Your Stomach**, is my experience with COVID-19's gastrointestinal rout, with the connection between gut and brain. Nothing I learned then or since has shed light on the mechanisms or consequences of the gut infection. Applying our intuition is all the more important here.

Chapter seven, **Time to Look Around**, reviews the medical and media context of what we see, what we know, and what we feel. The emphasis is on integration: to understand how these disjoint aspects of the pandemic could be different parts of the same system.

Chapter eight, **Future Visions**, returns to the microscopic. We take matters into our own hands and address the central battleground of the infection: our cells. What does it mean for a virus to breach a cell, and what tools in our arsenal can combat this?

Chapter nine, **Rethinking the Implausible**, takes this a step further: down to the level of molecules. Now, the issue is chemical, and the question becomes our control over our body's chemical and electrical systems.

Chapter ten, **Viral Fatigue**, steps beyond what is advertised as "the disease" to bring into focus the post-acute infection. The so-far ignored issue of post-viral infection is brought into focus. It is destined to come into focus since it can be debilitating, chronic, and widespread.

Chapter eleven, **Spirit**, moves beyond the body to ask for the virus's spiritual implications. Does it give us a sense of purpose, or are we a victim of its purpose? If health and healing exist beyond medicine and social policy, then how do we get there, and should we be working towards getting there now?

Chapter twelve, **Ecology Big and Small**, asserts that spirit when seen in the large is not the realm of deity but ecology. Certainly, the cosmos is home to the divine, but perhaps the virus's larger reality is a call to personal strength, a larger mind, and an awakening for individuals to control the future through the evolution of their thoughts.

The summary of chapter thirteen, **Consilience of Reason and Emotion**, proposes these pieces have a common future. Consilience is the unity of separate fields—science and the humanities in particular. Resolving COVID-19 will not end all the conflicts, but the conflicts inflamed by COVID-19 will only resolve along with the fundamental conflicts that underlie them.

Hypnosis

The world we see is an illusion, and there are participants in it who see our world differently. Our illusion doesn't define reality.

Microbes see a world we could not possibly imagine. The Greenland shark lives 500 years in a solitary world of boundless darkness. Forest trees have a community consciousness that decides when to make it rain. Chromosomes outlive our bodies following their own path of adaptation and evolution. The ecosystem as a whole follows a poly-rhythm of parts with durations ranging from chemical reactions to continental drift.

We've created machines allowing us to describe aspects we cannot see, but technology has also removed us from our environment. It's this less varied experience, not our knowledge of the details, that defines our consensual reality. What is "real" for each system is defined by what each interacts with, and the speed at which this happens.

Asking you to imagine a different reality is a small request. Imagining yourself to be in control, healthy, and aware means recognizing the degree to which you are not, but could be more in control, healthy, and aware. Is that really so much to ask? That's all that hypnosis does: ask you to imagine another reality to such a degree that you believe it.

> "Despite substantial variation in techniques among the numerous reports, patients treated with hypnosis experienced substantial benefits for many different medical conditions."
>
> — **James M. Stewart**, MD, from "Hypnosis in Contemporary Medicine" (Stewart, 2005)

Change

The world you see is the illusion we've agreed on. Most of the time we agree, as long as we don't look too closely. We don't ask what exactly is the smell of a rose because we can't answer this question. We get along by not asking "why?"

When things don't "get along" they change or disappear. Humans have created ecological crises in which this is happening in many quarters. How quickly we can change our relationship with our environment will determine which relationships find a new balance and which relationships disappear.

Human inclinations have shown little change, but then evolution is driven by necessity not by intention. There are too many simultaneous changes that need to be made for any single strategy to drive an ecology.

This work is partly an exposition and partly a reprogramming. In each chapter, the text explains the guided visualizations in the way that descriptions describe paintings. In the guided visualizations you're asked to become the story I'm telling not as a reader or a listener, but as a participant. To really be there. Like art, hypnotism reframes your traumatic history providing new space for your character to change.

In all these visualizations I am leading you to a visceral connection of your mind's intention and to a new experience. This may seem foreign at first, but it comes with practice. Practice both in relaxing the critical mind and in unleashing the creative one.

Use sleep and dreams. Listen to these inductions before going to bed, or before going into a contemplative situation and let them brew and steep. The visualizations might reappear in your dreams but, more likely, they will color your dreams. That's all you're aiming for: to have your intentions considered by the subconscious part of your mind that manages your affairs.

Chapter two's visualization, **Nose and Throat**, is our first exploration into heightened awareness. Relaxation is your first goal. Being aware of your breath is a primary means to attain relaxation.

Chapter three's **Your Lymphatic System** asks you to trace in your body a system you're never felt or, if you have felt it with a swelling here or there, to put it together as a whole. Recognize that there is an essential part of you that you have never seen, but that you can see and enhance.

Chapter four's **Unwinding the Negative** is a call to a sense of positive action. The combination of foreboding and misinformation has led to mass anxiety with a self-reinforcing effect. By pushing hard on the rudder, *Unwinding the Negative* seeks to exit this tailspin.

Chapter five's **Airways** leads you down your esophagus and into your lungs as a participant, not a victim. The whole mechanical, Western medical approach is victim-based. This is dangerous, unjustified, and ridiculous.

Chapter six presents **The Gut Part I-Stomach** for those who want greater upper gastrointestinal awareness. There are massive connections between our minds and our G.I. tract. You know of this, but you are scarcely a participant in it. You can be. You just need to pay attention.

Chapter seven, **The Voyage**, calls for emotional balance. It is the emotions that reside in the gut through the gut's effect on hormones and neurotransmitters. Saddle an awareness of the gut and take the reins of emotion in order to educate your immune system.

In chapter eight's visualization, **Membrane Locksmith**, I take you to the abstract level of your membranes, the front line in your defense against infection. I suggest the unreasonable idea that you have the power to control individual cells of your body. Unreasonable as it may be, it is demonstrably true.

Mind and Molecules, in chapter nine, continues building your relationship with your microscopic awareness through the concept of current. These currents provide the energy that supports your chemistry. You experience current as energy in your tissues. Let's call it by its oriental name: chi.

With chapter ten's **The Harmony of the Microbes**, we move past the acute phase to reconstruction, or so we hope. Chronic viral fatigue does not affect everyone, but for those who are affected, the gut seems to hold the key. These are the microbes we want to harmonize, those cells of your body that COVID-19 has thrown into disarray.

Chapter eleven's **Spirit and Reason** is the first of our two spiritual excursions. This first excursion opens you to a greater beyond, beyond your body and into a land of personal meaning. Here resides your purpose and motivation; the reason for healing and patience.

Our final journey, chapter twelve's **Ecology**, is an invitation to experience yourself as part of a larger system. That's all ecology is: systems. They're layered over and around each other, sometimes parallel and at other times intersecting.

You're part of it. As small as you may think you are, you are not small because these systems are not entirely stable, and that's what your mind is for: to guide these systems. You are the intelligence in the machine.

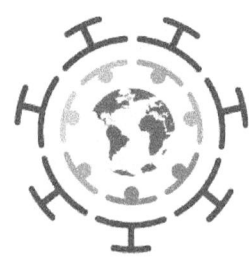

2 – Hypnosis for the New Flu

The quackery of medicine, and other things to boost your immunity.

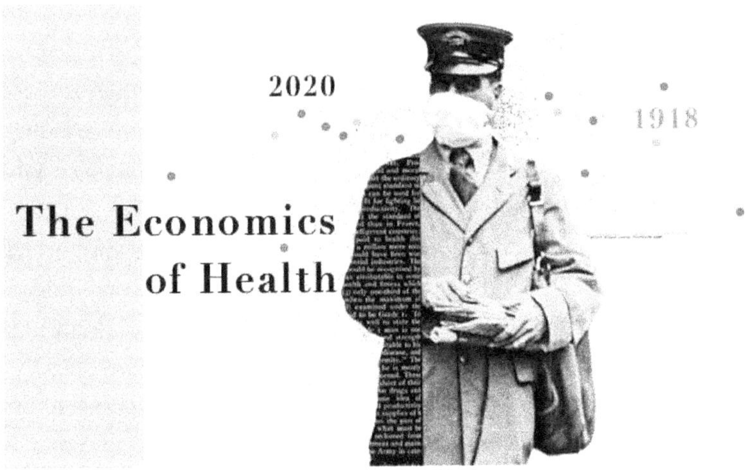

"That which does not kill us, makes us stronger."
— **Friedrich Nietzsche**

What The News Says

The official name of the coronavirus is SARS-CoV-2. "SARS" for Severe Acute Respiratory Syndrome. "CoV" for coronavirus. And "2" for the second to be given this name. Initially discovered in China in the fall of 2019, it was first identified in North American in January of 2020. It had been around for some previous months, probably on many continents, but not recognized for what it was.

At first, mass media discussions of the impending COVID-19 illness focused on the lack of medical recourse largely ignoring natural ways to boost one's health, resistance, and immunity. Even months later there was little talk about maintaining, improving, or assuring one's health, as if everyone was expected to feel victimized.

A March 10th article in the *New York Times*, titled, "Can I Boost My

Immune System," (Pope, 2020) encouraged boosting immune function with lower stress and improved sleep habits. There was quiet mention of earlier controlled studies that had shown long-term supplementation of vitamin D lowered respiratory infections by 40% in the elderly, while zinc supplements lowered respiratory infections in children by 45%.

A buffet of promising dietary and herbal supplements, without numbers or recommendations, advised moderation and a healthy attitude. It was another month before health care sites and mainstream journals—responding to a ground-swell of interest—started recommending supplements of vitamins C and D as well as zinc, and a few others (Martinson, 2020).

Nuanced approaches and long-term strategies seem beyond government, hospitals, and doctors. These authorities consider themselves "responsible," which means they're responsive, which means no one paid them to learn, prepare, train, or react on a moment's notice. Being bureaucratically constrained, they cannot provide a quick and accurate response to an unprecedented situation—as should be plainly obvious. Only you can learn and act on your own behalf, immediately, and in your best interests.

Everybody's Doing It

COVID-19 spreads like a bad flu against which we have no resistance (Rettner, 2020). Every year, variants of the influenza virus sweep the world and half a million die. No one makes a big deal about it. It's just a fact of life. But this similarity is deceiving.

The flu is largely pulmonary, and not everyone is susceptible to it; most of us have some resistance. In addition, the flu is somewhat predictable in its effects. It is an equal-opportunity infector, though weaker immune systems are more likely to develop more severe symptoms.

COVID-19 is not the flu and it's not strictly pulmonary. In fact, COVID-19 is not a disease, it's an infection. A disease is defined as a dysfunction or impaired structure or tissue associated with specific symptoms. COVID-19 is not this.

SARS-CoV-2 creates an infection that can disrupt many tissues and organs in the body. The specificity we ascribe to disease combines what we've been taught to experience with how medicine has divided the body into specialties.

The SARS-CoV-2 virus actually doesn't care what tissues it invades as long as it can reproduce itself. That's determined by its biochemistry, not our body functions. The symptoms we manifest are our reaction to it.

Most illnesses reflect our body's immune response, not the action of the infectious agent. Quite a few infections cause no illness at all, and we're not even aware that we are infected. We don't have many different immune responses, so these various diseases that do trigger our immune response in a particular organ will manifest the same symptoms in us. It's often our immune response—or our unsuccessful immune response—that is the most threatening to us.

The SARS-CoV-2 virus is not specifically pulmonary, it simply reaches the lungs first. In some cases, it gets a foothold in the gastrointestinal tract first. This happened to me. I'm sure I got it from my son and his school environment, and I both breathed it in and ingested it through food. But it manifested in my gut and never in my lungs. In any case, these are just starting points. Once inside the body it can invade cells almost anywhere, causing any sort of damage, reaction, or disruption. What it affects in a person seems to depend more on the person than on the virus.

Given that this virus is not that unusual, it's surprising that our reaction to it is so unusual. The virus is one of a dozen corona viruses whose other family members give us little more than the common cold. This virus just seems to have gotten particularly lucky—from its point of view—in hitting on the right protein key making it ten to twenty times more efficient in entering our cells. This has to be seen as a matter of luck for the virus since it did not evolve to infect humans but rather to infect other species.

The viruses efficient means of breaching our cellular membranes results in collateral damage to our cellular functions. One small change in the viruses chemistry can change it from benign to virulent. For the most part, the virus is simply hijacking a membrane protein in order to enter the cell. Unfortunately, it's a crucial protein called ACE2 and disrupting its function can cause chaos, organ dysfunction, and cellular starvation.

COVID-19 is sufficiently new that no one is immune and everyone is susceptible. This, it seems, is what makes it epidemiologically different from the flu. The viruses symptoms are minor or absent in over 80% of cases, and serious to severe in under 20% of cases.

The virus's benign effect makes it more dangerous because it's transmitted by people who don't even know they have it. A malign virus would be sequestered both by quarantine and by the victim's inability to move about, but this virus spreads widely before it reaches those who react the worst. From the virus's point of view, the people who get sick represent its failure. It doesn't want us to get ill; it wants us to thrive in order to spread everywhere.

There are some claims that COVID-19 is less contagious than influenza. This is unclear, because we don't know how many people are infected. We say the flu is too contagious to contain, but this is really a statement of our indifference to its consequences.

> "Asymptomatic transmission is the Achilles' heel of COVID-19 pandemic control through the public-health strategies we have currently deployed"
>
> — **Gandhi, Yokoe, & Havlir** (2020)

No one seems to be sure just how to contain COVID-19, but the idea seems to be that if its spread can be prevented, then it will die out before it infects everyone. This seems unlikely. The flu doesn't die out. Maybe one strain does, but others follow. And the reason the flu dies out may have more to do with the weather than anything we're doing. I had always thought cold weather makes humans more susceptible, but it turns out that warm weather that makes most virus weaker. So, if it was always cold, we might always have the flu—just one strain after another.

Another question being asked is whether annual mutations are going to give us one corona virus after another. There are dozens of them, we do see this one mutating, and this is what viruses always do. Perhaps the idea is that corona viruses don't mutate as fast as influenza so that the next one won't be right on its heels. Or perhaps, the mutations will be sufficiently minor that the immunity we acquire this year will give us protection against the strain that evolves next year.

Many people are hoping that once this first corona variant sweeps the world, enough people will have developed immunity that subsequent variants won't reach epidemic proportions. They'll just flare up and go out. The trouble is, lacking any history to go on, no one can predict how different or how lethal the next strain of the virus will be.

Exposure

It has always been my impression that one can get a greater or lesser case of something, and your degree of illness depends on these aspects:

- Nature of the illness
- Quantity to which you're exposed
- Strength of your immunity

The nature of the illness is fixed at whatever it is, and, because it's a virus, Western medicine is largely in the dark. Viral illnesses make understood bacterial infections seem like a walk in the park.

Perhaps the worst advice I first heard about what to do if you feel ill is to see your doctor. It seems like no one has a clue anymore about how to take care of themself.

No one has indicated that seeing your doctor will result in anything other than some reassuring words or a ticket to the hospital for an IV drip, stress, contagion, co-infection, general chaos, and emergency intervention if you're lucky.

The wisdom in calling the doctor—that is calling as in phoning, not seeing them in person—is that they'll have up-to-date information and, if they know your history, they may know your risks better than you do.

Nevertheless, the first thing you should do is get informed. Familiarize yourself with prevention strategies and do that now, not when you feel ill! Getting set up for recovery at home should be a first, proactive response so that you don't have to go milling about in public when you're ill (Barclay & Scott, 2020).

Then, there is the issue of the quantity to which you're exposed. I wonder about this. When I first started writing, no one was talking about this. For what I can tell, it's implied that you either get a full dose or you don't catch it at all. No one was asking if there was a possibility of having a limited infection if you had a limited exposure. There is no test for the quantity to which you've been exposed, not to mention that there few available COVID-19 tests for anyone, anyway.

On the one hand, pathogens multiply exponentially, so that, whether you start with two or two hundred thousand, it takes only a handful of doubling cycles before the infection is firmly established. In spite of this, it can take up to five days for symptoms to appear.

But things are not so simple. The rate at which the pathogen invades is balanced by the rate at which your system responds, which depends on where in your body the virus is establishing itself and how you're responding to it. And while you cannot control the pathogen's reproductive rate, you can give it a less hospitable home and mount a stronger resistance to it.

I'm now writing at the end of May, and I'm just starting to hear this mentioned. On May 19th, Eric Levenson of CNN reported, "Growing evidence suggests that COVID-19 infection, like with other illnesses, is related to prolonged time exposed to the virus. The longer you stay in an environment that may contain the virus, the higher the risk of getting sick." Now, finally, the CDC suggests that 15 minutes of close exposure could be used as a basis for contagion. Of course, this is a very rough rule-of-thumb.

We're told that infection in the upper respiratory tract is far milder than infection lower down in the lungs. We're told that wearing a face mask—as opposed to a respirator—will offer little to no protection. How about breathing through your nose? Limiting infections to your upper respiratory tract is the reason you have a nose, see Gwen Lawrence's "Breathing" (Lawrence, 2020), yet many people are mouth-breathers.

In my town of Victoria, BC, mouth-breathing is a fashion—I think it's Canadian. I regularly count mouth-breathers when I'm in public and the rate appears to be over fifty percent. People should be advised to shut their mouths. Which brings me to my third item: your immunity. See "6 Immune System Busters & Boosters" (WebMD Medical Reference, 2019).

Four Easy Steps

- Step one: You don't have the virus. At first, that's everybody.
- Step two: You've been infected but you don't know. There are no symptoms. For many people, that's the end of it.
- Step three: You're infected. You have symptoms and they're getting worse.
- Step four: You're seriously ill. 15 - 20% of those with symptoms get

seriously ill and need medical attention. Most have existing health conditions. Up to 20% of this smaller population die. (Richardson et al., 2020).

In an amazing reflection on the workings of the US health care system, people who felt they were at step three and went to the hospital suspecting they had the virus were told to go home and return only if they became seriously ill. That is, health care was only being made available at stage four, where it had a limited, positive effect. Hospital resources focused on those needing intensive care, half of whom perished in spite of it.

On March 31st, Dr. Roger Seheult, a pulmonologist and emergency room doctor broadcasting medical updates through the Medcram.com website, said the medical system was "doing a lot of nothing (at stage three) when the immune systems needs a lot of help."

There are many kinds of immunity. The two basic kinds are immunity from infection, which I'll call resistance, and the response of the immune system to infection, which I'll call immune response. Neither of these involves medical intervention; they both can be enhanced and supported. The emergency medical system provides no proactive support for your immune system.

Immunity

Few to no one in the mainstream press is talking about how to build, maintain, or support your immunity. Maybe the topic is considered boring, intellectual, or not sufficiently sensational. All the talk is about contagion and death, and none of the talk is about resistance.

This strikes me as so abysmally stupid that it almost makes me want to root for the virus. Perhaps the real molecular receptor site of the COVID-19 virus is the stupid molecule. From an evolutionary point of view, that idea has some merit.

The Western approach to increasing immunity is taking a pill. Unfortunately, Western pharmacists have not settled the question of what pills are the best immune boosters, so we'll have to go with folk medicine.

Vitamin C

Linus Pauling endorsed Vitamin C and won two Nobel Prizes for his work—

one was the Peace Prize—but he was such a contentious character that Vitamin C remains bush medicine to most doctors. Even so—because of Pauling—everyone believes it works at what Pauling would consider a minimal dose. Incidentally, because of this belief Walmart quickly and entirely sold out of Vitamin C.

It is said that you can't overdose on Vitamin C, so megadoses may not hurt you, but it is not entirely benign. Large doses, above 2 or 3 grams per day, commonly cause diarrhea and have led to pseudogout (a form of arthritis), pancreatitis (a potentially dangerous inflammation of the pancreas), and kidney stones (Briggs, 1984)

One gram per day is pretty standard though it's above the minimum requirement. Pauling took between 3 and 20 grams per day; reports vary. Vitamin C is ascorbic acid. It costs almost nothing and, through to the end of March, no one in the mainstream press had mentioned it, or any other immune boosters, for that matter.

Pauling endorsed Vitamin C because it prevents oxidation within the cell, and oxidizing chemicals are a destructive by-product of cellular respiration. Pauling's theory was that getting as much vitamin C into and around the cell would help neutralize dangerous oxidants which would prevent illnesses of all kinds. It is now known that oxidative stress leads to many illnesses.

I am a system theorist, which means I always try to look at the whole system. It does not surprise me that Pauling's theory was lacking. It turns out that "the use of antioxidants to treat various clinical disorders may not be as simple as it originally sounded" (Koren, Kohen, & Ginsburg, 2010).

While oxidants are dangerous to the stability of other molecules and to processes within the cell, the cell understands this and deals with it. More importantly, and more wisely, the cell uses these dangerous oxidants for other purposes; they are not garbage. Oxidants are moved out of the cell and into or onto red (Koren et al., 2010) and white (Bolin, Guerra, Nascimento, & Otton, 2012) blood cells where they perform essential functions. This process is just starting to be understood, so there is no conclusion about the full benefits and risks of taking supplementary antioxidants, like vitamin C.

When it comes to the use of vitamins of all kinds I believe one should listen to one's body and follow its direction. Speaking only for myself, I have not noticed vitamin C to help in my recovery from illness. I have no scientific support for this, it's just the evidence my body presents. I am uncertain about vitamin C's effect on my resistance.

Vitamin D and Zinc

There are cellular biological arguments in support of boosting vitamin D and zinc levels to help fend off the effects of SARS-CoV-2 within the cell. My personal experience was that taking a high level of zinc supplements, around 100 mg/day, felt fortifying. Lower doses did not. Zinc comes largely from the diet. There is much anecdotal evidence being shared between doctors that zinc is helpful in the treatment of COVID-19, and zinc supplements are being widely endorsed.

Vitamin D is both ingested and produced by your body in reaction to sunlight. Also, different races product different amounts with the lighter skinned races producing more of it. The arguments for vitamin D are also biochemical, but the levels of it differ widely as do, I suspect, people's reaction to vitamin D supplements.

Whereas zinc is a mineral, vitamin D is both an exogenous and endogenous protein. You can buy supplements of both but they should not be seen as similar. I found that taking the maximum suggested dosage of 100 mcg/day (4,000 IU) of vitamin D weakened my constitution and soured my mood. I am taking 25 mcg/day (1,000 IU), which is slightly above the recommended intake of 10-20 mcg/day.

There is much anecdotal evidence for vitamin D's role in boosting resistance (DeNoon, 2020) for which I find little conclusive scientific support. A 2017 report in the British Medical Journal (Martineau et al., 2017) concluded "Vitamin D supplementation was safe and it protected against acute respiratory tract infection overall."

A 2011 study in *Experimental Biology and Medicine* concluded, "At this time it would be premature to suggest that vitamin D might be useful to improve host resistance to TB, influenza or any other infectious organism." Note that this is a carefully worded sentence that says nothing. However, their use of the vague word "premature" seems to leave a bad taste in one's mouth.

Herbals

There are many herbal remedies; we've all got our favorites. Herbals can be just as powerful as prescription medicines. They have side effects and can be dangerous. I'll only mention elderberries. They're cheap, powerful, relatively safe, and normally they're widely available. They're an ingredient in all sorts of herbals, from tinctures to throat lozenges.

I purchased a cup of the dried berries which I boiled into a thick decoction and to which I added a quarter of a cup of whisky—it was the only alcohol I had around. Before I got sick I had been putting a teaspoon of this decoction into my tea. You can find recipes on the Web. It should be noted that raw elderberries contain toxins and must be processed.

This addition felt fortifying and enervating. I go by what feels right. For little more than the love of berries I give it credit for mitigating my symptoms. There is a lot of anecdotal evidence in support of this, and some science-based evidence as well.

However, the indications are that while helpful for resistance, elderberries may be unhelpful for recovery, and I did get that feeling. I continued taking this as a supplement for a week after I got ill, but then stopped. Maybe it was the whiskey, but I have not yet gone back to it and I don't feel drawn to.

There are many other herbal supplements, some with science-based endorsement and many without. I'm drawn more to species than science—I love mushrooms—but each person to his or her own. In general, herbals contain mysterious agglomerations of inscrutable molecules which are "natural," while science-based formulas and experiments can only deal with reduced, simplified, unnatural and energetically denuded substances (which is a whole other discussion).

Sleep

The other interesting immune booster you'll never hear about is sleep. See "How sleep can boost your body's immune response," in *Medical News Today*. I'll bet that if you stopped what you were doing, avoided stress, and got ten hours of sleep every day, then your immunity would improve dramatically. I have so much vitriol from being denied my dreams in order to get to school—and that includes graduate school—that I'll just refer you to the literature and move on to hypnosis.

Suffice it to say that getting more sleep is not only the most important way to build both resistance and strengthen immune response, but it is also the key to solving most of your life's problems. At least it is if you use sleep as a way to engage and not a means to disengage. For more on that topic, see my books on sleep and dreaming (Stoller, 2019a; Stoller, 2019b).

> "Neglect sleep, and you are deciding to perform a genetic engineering manipulation on yourself each night, tampering with the nucleic alphabet that spells out your daily health story."
>
> — **Matthew Walker** (2017), from *Why We Sleep: The New Science of Sleep and Dreams*

Hypnosis and Illness

The connection between hypnosis and illness lies in the field of psycho-neuro-immunology. I'm not sure if I love or hate this word. On the good side, it's self explanatory, at least if you're somewhat familiar with the field. On the bad side, it's another highbrow denial-of-service attack on our autonomy. Granted, this could be a big study; but it has a large do-it-yourself aspect which Western medicine should keep its grubby paws off of.

Psycho-neuro-immunology is the interface between your mind, your nervous system, and your immune system. It's a potentially huge field because it includes all three, but it could also remain marginal if no one is able to make sense of it.

It's now well established that your mental state affects your chemical balance, and your chemical balance influences your immune system. The most general mechanism that affects your balance is stress, so it's somewhat odd that few health practitioners have recognized how little they know about stress, or have made any effort to learn. Hypnotists are the exception because relaxation —one aspect of stress reduction—has always been the key ingredient.

Stress flips your nervous system into a contracted, focused, and vigilant state. The opposite of stress—which we can call relaxation only if you recognize just how broadly it can apply—returns a system to its balanced and recuperative state. Hypnosis works in medicine by deepening and broadening one's resting state.

There's more to the resting state than rest. Everything you do that isn't fighting, freezing, fleeing, fainting, or overexerting yourself is done in your resting state. That includes reasoning, thinking, learning, digesting, reproducing, growing, healing, and enjoying yourself. Each of these activities involves a balanced dynamic that's only possible when these activities can be given your full, relaxed attention, without fear or hesitation. Stress is antithetical to this state of flow.

Correct exercise is also done in a mental resting state, a homeostatic state that you can maintain for long periods of time. Even extreme exercise puts you in a zone of mental quiet and physical balance. Athletes know this and aim for it because optimal performance exists in this relaxed state of action.

This is what hypnosis does: it helps you put into direct focus those things you may be only marginally conscious of. The result could be improved performance in almost anything, from thinking to feeling to being to acting. But what's relevant here is your immune system.

The Immune Response

Unfortunately for the curious, your immune system operates almost entirely on a molecular level. There are few gross measurements we can make. In addition, it's involved throughout your body and, like the Men In Black, it keeps a low profile. It's the National Security Agency of your system, a central intelligence agency whose main task is collecting information and stimulating your immune response.

I think about the immune system as having receptive and active parts. There's more to it, but I think this is where a hypnotherapy program should start. The receptive part involves the collection of information about what's happening in your body. In this aspect, your immune system is benign and the issue is how to heighten sensitivity.

The active part of the immune system involves its immune response, and your immune response is anything but benign. Your immune response can kill you. Here, the role of hypnosis is managerial.

The immune response is biological, neurological, and chemical. It enlists white blood cells to attack invaders, chemicals to trigger inflammation and perfusion, and neural signals to trigger a wide-area sympathetic (tensing) response.

It involves the release of neurotransmitters and hormones that reorient cells throughout the body. This is mysterious stuff. Don't let anyone fool you into thinking we've got it figured out. As the neurophysiologist Jerry Lettvin told me, "Hormones are chemicals that no one understands."

It seems possible that relaxation, in some deep sense, could improve both the receptive and active aspects of the immune system. For the moment, I focus on the receptive aspect.

Who Knows About Interoception?

I'm writing a book of hypnotic inductions to improve one's internal functions. I began this project when I made the connection between hypnosis, brainwave training, and heart-rate variability. Let me give you the elevator pitch.

Hypnosis can change your brainwaves. It can also equilibrate the neuronal control of your cardio-pulmonary system. This system has been found to be an indicator of the tone of your sympathetic nervous system which, in turn, is connected to your immune response. My idea is to cut to the chase: use hypnosis to potentiate immune sensitivity and response.

At first, people looked at brainwaves as a signature of the hypnotic state. Then, I noticed that one's brainwave state could be guided by directive hypnosis. This seemed to be on the tip of other people's tongues but no one was saying it. My neurofeedback colleagues were uninterested in their client's mentation, and my hypnotherapeutic colleagues couldn't care less about cerebral electrical emanations. So it remains to this day. I only know of two people interested in this cross-over field: me and Ron Pekala, who's at the Coatesville Veterans Affairs Medical Center in Pennsylvania.

The lack of interest is almost a joke, but there you have it; very few of us have the right combination of skills. I publish articles about neurofeedback in the hypnosis trade journals. I see psychologists publishing on the same topic in psychological trade journals. We both admonish our colleagues that establishing neural correlates with our work in hypnosis and psychology will be essential. So far, we've gotten about as much response as epidemiologists warning about virus preparedness.

Hypnosis for the Nose and Throat

I've been creating hypnotic inductions for various body systems. I aim to create a comprehensive library covering basic functions. So far, I've prepared inductions for liver function, peripheral circulation, small intestine, body polarity, body frequencies, body resonances, and heart and lung. At the end of this chapter is an induction called *Nose and Throat* that aims to improve the function of the tissues in your nose and throat.

Nose and Throat is a sensory exploration: a combination of imagination and heightened awareness. The object is to be mindful about your breath and responsive to the sensations in your throat and maxillary sinuses. Beyond that, my hope is that through creative visualization you will gain some control over the autonomic functions of blood flow, mucus production, and immune response in the sinus and throat tissues.

This is an extrapolation of the observation that hypnotized patients can exsanguinate the blood supply to warts and diminish internal bleeding during surgery, abilities that are only explainable if there is a greater measure of control than is consciously available and considered possible.

Not wanting to stop at the implausible, I explore the possibility that you can gain awareness within these tissues, and gain greater control of them. If you suck warm water into your nose, you'll notice it feels quite uncomfortable. If you add a half teaspoon of salt to a half cup of warm water and suck it into your nose it feels very comfortable. You have sensory nerves on the surface of your sinus tissues that enable you to discriminate in ways you have never explored. What else can you do?

Nose and Throat is the first of the proactive tools offered for your defense against COVID-19. Listen to this induction repeatedly with the aim of becoming more sensitive to what your throat and sinuses are telling you. Use your mind to create images and to experience feelings. Focus on creating a new awareness of things you didn't have an awareness of before. It's my hope that with heightened sensitivity a stronger immune response will develop in these tissues.

Hypnotic Session 1

Nose and Throat audio file at: https://www.mindstrengthbalance.com/covid19-illness-illumination/

Nose and Throat

Nose and Throat is a hypnotic induction that requires your full attention. Do not listen to this hypnotic visualization if you are driving a car, operating machinery, or doing anything that requires your attention.

The purpose of this induction is to help you get in greater touch with the sensations, the signals, and the awareness you have in these tissues. With things you might nor normally experience, or overlook as incidental, imaginary, or unnecessary. For you to take a deeper look, and get a deeper sense of these areas of your body during your normal course of events: breathing, swallowing, licking your lips, chewing your food. And in abnormal courses of events, such as sneezing, coughing, such that you come into greater allegiance with the sensations that you feel and the sensations that come over you, like twitches or itches.

And we're here to release those tensions, so that you don't have to react to every sensation. Allay any tensions or any discomfort by relaxing the tissues. Perfusing them with moisture.

Begin this exercise by relaxing. By finding a comfortable position where you can close your eyes and start to imagine sensations and visualize pictures, where you won't be disturbed, and you have nothing else to do but focus on your breath.

Start by simply taking a breath. Simply inhale… and then exhale…

Inhale… and exhale.

Imagine the front of your forehead relaxing as if there was a hand brushing back over your ears, down the sides of your head, down the back of your neck as if someone was petting you, as if you were a cat and you close your eyes and you purr. Across your brow, over the side of your head, and down the back of your neck. Focus on the sensation.

And let that feeling of relaxation that goes over and down your neck continue down your back and over your shoulders, and down your arms to your hands where it makes your hands warmer, and down your back to your hips and your waist where it makes your body warmer, and down your legs, over your thighs, through your knees, through your bones to your ankles to your feet where your tensions relax and your tissues get warmer.

Now, as you start to take the next breath, focus on your nostrils and be aware of the cooler air that moves past your nostrils as you inhale through your nose, and imagine that you're following that air into your nose, and imagine it's as if going into a dark room, but it's not all that dark, there is light, it's faint light. And the tissues in your nose are in a hollow chamber, the sinuses in the front of your head, and they're rather large, such as you might encircle by holding your thumb and forefinger together.

As the air enters your nostrils, into your sinuses, it tumbles in a kind of chaotic turbulence brushing across the surface of your membranes, sensitive skin throughout your sinuses. You can feel the space behind your nose and when you inhale it tingles. And there are chambers leading up and leading back into your skull of smaller rooms with smaller spaces and these chambers are lined with cells that can smell, and you can smell the air that you inhale.

And as you continue to inhale, the air goes back down your throat to small openings at the base of your sinuses into the top of your throat. Your can feel the air passing through those passageways. And imagine at the top of your throat the soft tissues at the back or your pallet which are moist with saliva as the air passes them, and becomes moist itself on its way down into your lungs.

And as you release your breath, and the air comes up, out of your nose, notice that the air is warm and the air is moist, and recognize that the air you breath in has more oxygen in it, and as it goes into you lungs you extract that, and when you exhale you have put in its place carbon dioxide so that the air you breath out is different, and you can sense that, and you really can sense that through different sensors at different places in your system.

Now, with the next breath, open your mouth and inhale through your mouth, and feel the air tumble back behind your lips, behind your teeth, into the cavity left between your tongue and your pallet. And notice your teeth as if you had a search light inside your mouth that rotated around to illuminate your teeth from the inside.

Starting at the left, your upper teeth from your molars to the front incisors back to the right and the rear, back to your rear right molars and back to the lower right molars, beside your tongue, beneath your tongue, moving to the front, your lower incisors, to the left, your lower left molars. And your tongue, which you don't feel when it's resting, you can feel now, a large, muscular tissue that is part of you, that is sensitive in movement, taste, temperature, and humidity. And follow this tongue back behind your teeth, down into your throat where it's anchored.

And as the air passes your tongue it cascades into the back of the throat, where your Eustachian tubes come, where you tonsils are, your adenoids are. Tissues that protect you from infection, that regularly swell, and sometimes your throat is dry and sometimes you have a tickle in your throat.

Relax. Relax your tongue, relax your tissues. And make that connection between the back of your palate, your tongue, your lips, your mouth, and your sinuses as if they're all one large tract which do different things: sensing gases, sensing tastes, secreting saliva, chewing food, swallowing food, releasing the air from your ears.

And lower down into your voice box, into your vocal cords which stand like sentinels through which the air passes, and relax your vocal cords, let your throat extend, let it widen and soften. And if there is any inflammation from any irritation, any swelling, anywhere in your sinuses, in your mouth, in your gums, just relax those feelings, which may be real or imaginary, and imagine the blood of your system naturally, nutritively, cleaning, supplying, and supporting the tissues, the skin, the membranes.

And imagine the mucus whose job it is to transport, like a conveyor belt, dust and debris to keep moist and to make moist air that needs to be inhaled and exhaled, and how your body provides that moisture from your stores of liquid in your blood and plasma, from the food you eat and the liquid you drink, to keep your mouth, nose, throat, and tissues healthy.

Breathe deeply. Take a breath: inhale… exhale… and in the last part of this exercise I'd like you to imagine that you can breathe with just one nostril, and it may be possible, or it may just be that you feel more breath in one nostril, but imagine that you could open your left sinus and open your left nostril, and close your right nostril and sinus so that as you inhale through your nose more air comes in the left side. And exhale.

And switch now, opening up the right side, enlarging your right nostril, sensitizing your right sinus. And inhaling through what feels to be your right side. And relax now, and exhale.

Inhale… exhale…

And you might continue this into your lungs thinking the left lung inflates and then the right lung inflates, inhaling through your left nostril, inflating your right lung. Inhaling through your right nostril, inflating your left lung so that you have a sense of control and awareness of the air and the tissues.

And now relax and let this exercise go. Breathing calming, breathing into your relaxed body, breathing fully wholly and naturally. Feeling comfortable. Feeling clear and balanced, moist and comfortable.

3 – Hypnosis for Your Lymphatic System

Your most important system operates outside of your awareness.

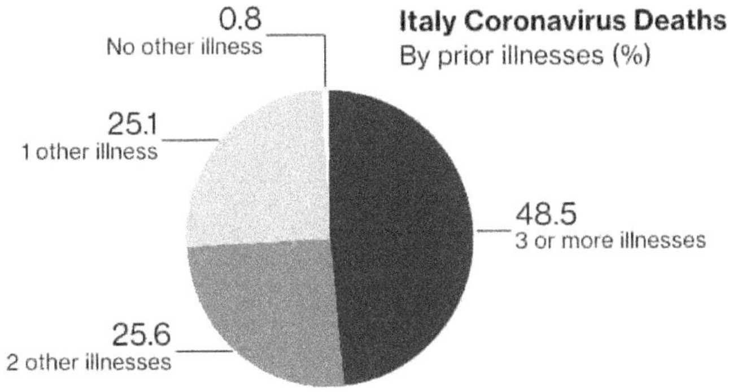

Source: ISS Italy National Health Institute, March 17, 2020 sample.

"The world is but a canvas for our imagination."
— **Henry David Thoreau**

Immunity and Mortality

It's hard to get good statistics from hospital reports because hospitals make no attempt to generalize, they attempt to treat each patient in a manner that will generate the best outcome. On top of that, different countries have different healthcare systems, and different population profiles. Early data coming out of China and Italy showed tentative trends, some of which grew stronger and are now recognized as indicative of the illness in general and not only the populations of those countries.

China has a high percentage of smokers, most of which are men, but the initial observation that the most severe cases affected the lungs of men was not due to smoking. The infection was transmitted largely through the air, hence infection started mostly in the lungs, and men have weaker immune systems than women. It was natural to assume, though it was not yet known so clearly, that having compromised pulmonary health strongly correlated with having a more severe case of the infection.

Italy's data, which was more transparent and more reliable, became available by the end of March. It clearly showed aging men were at higher risk, but, more importantly, those with compromised health constituted over 99% of the deaths. Italy was the second country to experience a crushing caseload, after China, partly because of where the virus happened to land next, and partly because of the large elderly proportion of the Italian population.

Italians are known for their friendly, physical nature and their disdain for authority. Characteristics that are now killing them. The necessity of social distancing was not yet recognized, and the idea was foreign to Italians. In a post on Instagram nine days before he tested positive, Nicola Zingaretti typified the Italian attitude by saying: "Let's not lose our habits, we can't stop Milan and Italy."

The Italian disease specialist Dr. Giovanni Guaraldi commented, "Initially, people do not really understand the message. We closed the schools but still people were gathering with one another… We need to be clear, the only way to protect against the spread of the epidemic is stay at home and try not to meet other people." The majority of patients who tested positive for the virus didn't require a trip to the hospital, he noted.

Even if all cases were being counted, Italy is the EU country with the highest percentage of elderly, and the elderly have a higher mortality rate. As the previous graph indicates, most of those dying are already ill and—in Italy at this time—unable to get adequate support.

If the actual mortality rate is 3.5%, as in Wuhan, China—which was the best guess at the time—and only 0.02% of healthy infected people are dying, then the actual mortality rate of the healthy population is 0.07%, which is about the same as the mortality rate of influenza in a previously exposed population. But we don't have a previously exposed population, which accounts for part of the higher mortality.

Italy's mortality rate climbed to 7%, but this was not representative of the whole population. Only the most serious cases were being counted, of which a higher percentage died. As the Italian hospitals were overwhelmed, the reported high mortality in conjunction with the crippled healthcare system drew world attention and incited varying degrees of world panic. This was at a time when public responses were just being considered at social, political, and economic levels. With the prospect of such high mortality rates, all parties could agree the potential for damage was serious, but different parties were prioritizing damage differently.

The Politics of Illness

The basic dichotomy in government responses to the pandemic centered on which interests needed protection and at what cost: the health of individuals or the health of the economy? And of those individuals, which segments of the population would be given the most protection. And regarding the economy, which industries would be given the most financial support?

These questions were made more complicated because of the lack of data, the uncertainty of applying foreign data to domestic populations, and the hiding of information for political advantage. Two of the most important factors that went unrecognized were population density and the ratio of people to healthcare resources. It soon became evident, as the virus moved into the US population, that the most densely populated cities were a petrie dish for the spread of the virus.

It was not at first noticed by the public, but slowly became evident as the death toll rose, that poorer segments of the population were at greater risk because of the higher density of their neighborhoods, their less well-endowed healthcare systems, their less sanitary jobs, and their higher dependence on remaining in at-risk jobs. The virus exaggerated the segregation of the US population by class, race, income, and culture in a country already under stress due to the inequities of those categories.

Unfortunately, for the people in several countries including the US, the pandemic occurred in the midst of a large anti-science bias that developed in response to the threat of global warming. The climate debate triggered a host of divisive issues that devolved into rule by misinformation. The issue has become politicized with doubting parties rejecting everything scientific. In those countries where these factions have gained leadership positions, anti-science bias has led to a rejection of expert healthcare advice. Such is the case in the

US, Britain, Brazil, and Russia, as well as smaller countries where politics are governed by institutional economics.

Policies in some countries discounted the dire warnings of epidemiologists partly because of a disbelieve in science—it can be assumed from the start that politicians don't understand science—or because this advice threatened the popularity of the leading party.

In the US, for example, the political response was almost exclusively aimed at providing corporate support as the federal government raised the national debt by 60% in three months—from 4 to 6.6 trillion—to support the stock and bond markets.

Based on my calculation of the total amount of support disbursements as of June, made to each of the current 140 million US taxpayers, less than 1/10th of these funds went to citizens in the form of one-time, $1,200 per person stimulus checks issued to as compensation for the two-month mandatory quarantine. No additional government assistance went to hospitals or healthcare services.

The US political system routinely under-represents its working class, and the government's weak response to the pandemic amplified a collective feeling of victimization. This, along with deeply established racial prejudice and Donald Trump, a deranged president, started a fire in dry tinder as riots swept across the country. The spark was several separate murders of African Americans in police custody, but the tinder was layered more deeply.

Sleep

Sleep is an immune enhancer, and it may be the most effective thing you can do to boost your immunity. Its positive effect is documented in an article entitled "Sleep after Vaccination Boosts Immunological Memory," in a 2011 issue of *The Journal of Immunology* (Lange, Bollinger, Dimitrov, & Diekelmann, 2011). Another review article, "Sleep and Immune Function," appearing in a 2011 issue of *The European Journal of Physiology* (Besedovsky, Lange, & Born, 2012), reports that "during the sleep phase, immune cells at early stages of differentiation peak in peripheral blood and lymph nodes."

These low-level studies correlate sleep cycles with biochemical measures. They measure the effect of sleep on T-cell counts, protein-induced inflammation, and antibody concentrations. These complex, indirect effects don't tell us how much one's immunity improves due to improved sleep, but, based on the subjective experience of one's immunological state when sleep-deprived, the effect is substantial. It can't be overlooked that when you're ill, your body wants to sleep.

I believe you can enhance your body's recuperative efforts during sleep by deepening your interoceptive sense before sleeping. You can achieve this through imagining, sensing, and focusing on the tissues, organs, and processes. Do this by entering a trance state in which you achieve a deeper connection with these autonomic processes. This is not so far-fetched. An article titled "Neural Responses to Heartbeats Distinguish Self from Other During Imagination" demonstrates that one's neurology is affected by imagination (Babo-Rebelo, Buot, & Tallon-Baudry, 2019).

The Lymphatic System

The lymphatic system, distributed throughout your body, acts to remove debris and to maintain, enhance, and accelerate recovery from infection. 100 billion of your cells die each day, roughly 1/3 of one percent of your body weight. These cells are eaten, dissolved, and disassembled by macrophages, a type of white blood cell, that travels through your circulatory and lymphatic systems consuming objects.

In addition to involving the lymphatic system, the immune function also relies on the release of hormones by the central nervous system, the enteric nervous system surrounding your gut, and the actions of white blood cells produced in bone marrow and other locations throughout your body.

Your lymphatic system consists of a one-way network of vessels. It is not a circulatory system, and it is separate from your circulatory system. Along this network are located your lymph nodes, which are repositories for white blood cells. These nodes are clustered in your torso, around your neck, under your arms, in your chest, belly, and groin. These—and hundreds of smaller nodules throughout your body—form the outposts that become swollen as your first reaction to infection.

I've created a guided visualization that focuses on your lymphatic system. This visualization encourages your engagement at three levels. First, the level of awareness: to focus on the regions where your lymph nodes are located and

—to whatever extent possible—relax them. Second, the level of energizing these locations: using your imagination to enhance their sensitivity—as if lymph nodes have a conscious awareness and can report what they are aware of. And third, joining your consciousness to that of your lymph nodes: taking up arms with them in solidarity and support.

There is no success or failure in this exercise; you're simply expanding and enhancing your awareness of this physically small and biologically sensitive system. There is nothing you have to achieve. Aim simply to feel fortified, whole, and in-tune. Imagine you control a complicated machine for which these lymph nodes are self-contained, supporting elements. You manage a jungle of species, all contributing in their own way to the balance of your body's ecosystem.

Daydream Work

Listen to this visualization and retain the detached state that results from it. Become more attuned to your lymphatic system while in your normal aware state. In the same way that a highly fit person sees the world from an enhanced perspective—gaining the sensitivity of heightened sensation and balanced flow—I encourage you to gain that aware state of your lymph nodes.

You will gain a waking sensitivity toward the areas where your nodes are located. Just as you can move through space with a heightened balance and awareness of the location of your limbs, so you will expand your awareness to "think from your lymph nodes."

Active Dream Work

Listen to *Your Lymphatic System* before going to sleep to make space in your mind for unusual feelings with the intention of carrying these into the dream-space. What you learn will come to you through thoughts, images, and feelings.

Give yourself permission to move into new territory, and give yourself the time and comfort to get there. Recognize that enlisting your imagination engages your lymphatic system. You're taking an active role. You're no longer an incidental participant, and you will have new experiences.

Your dream-time knows no small-talk, it does not come to you, and it does not speak your language. You will need to act on your intention to recall your dreams if you want to become aware. You need to sleep long enough to complete your dream cycle and decompress gradually upon waking. Take the initiative.

There are techniques to enhance dreams and dream recall. They rely on sleeping deeply and getting enough sleep to enable you to wake and rouse naturally, without rush or distraction, from the contemplation of your dreams. You can oversleep, that's OK. Being groggy just brings sleep further into your waking life.

Refer to my book *The Path To Sleep, Exercises for an Ancient Skill* (Stoller, 2019a) to balance your sleep rhythms. Refer to my book *Becoming Lucid, Self-Awareness in Sleeping and Waking Life* (Stoller, 2019b) for a deeper understanding of your sleeping and waking states. These books are available online in print, digital, and audiobook formats.

Listen to the audio *Your Lymphatic System* before going to sleep each night for at least a week. Don't worry if you fall asleep during the process, or if you don't remember what's been said. You don't need to remember it. You can remain unattached and uninvested in thinking about anything. Let your mind wander in comfortable ways. You will change your thinking in subtle ways, and, more than that, there will be changes in what you feel.

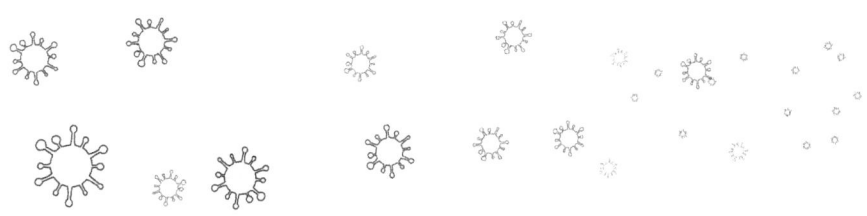

Hypnotic Session 2

Your Lymphatic System audio file at:
https://www.mindstrengthbalance.com/covid19-illness-illumination/

Your Lymphatic System

Your Lymphatic System is a hypnotic induction that requires your full attention. Do not listen to this hypnotic visualization if you are driving a car, operating machinery, or doing anything that requires your attention.

This is an imaginary exploration of your lymphatic system. It requires that you lie down and be warm. It's a difficult exploration because it's a complicated and subtle system. It has no beating heart, no central organ, no membrane that surrounds it. Unlike your blood, it has no simple function, and while your blood isn't really simple, it's simpler.

Prepare to lay down on a bed with a blanket you will put over yourself. You want to be warm. We're opening your body, and it needs to be warm inside where we're going. Better it is warmer than cooler, your lymphatic system likes heat because it likes blood, and your tissues open to circulation when they're warm.

And we'll use your hands, because hands have energy, and your lymphatic system is an energy system. It's all about information, surveillance, and response. Use your awareness and your sensations.

You'll place your hands over your abdomen, but not just anywhere, precisely here: your fingertips will touch your pubic bone at the base of your pelvis just above your genitals, and the palms of your hands will lie on the flat of your lower stomach, your thumbs touching and the sides of your hands above your groin area, at the edges of your gut. The heels of your palms will be just above the arc at the top of your large intestine which lies all the way at the back of your body, against your spine.

And we'll move your hands during this exploration, but they'll start here, over your lower abdomen—with the center of your palms over your small intestine—and they'll end here, when we reach the end of this journey.

If you're not lying down yet, lie down now. Make yourself most comfortable, and lay beneath a substantial blanket. Something heavy; something warm. And your arms are at your sides with your palms against your lower abdomen, and you would be looking at the ceiling, but you're not, because your eyes are closed. And you want to close them because this is a movie, and it's being projected on the backs of your eyelids, and you have to have a movie screen, or you can't see it.

Your head is comfortable. You're laying on a pillow or something else that supports your head and neck so you can relax your neck and your head won't roll to either side. And you can let your head sink further, and your neck relax, until it almost feels like there's nothing holding your vertebrae together at all.

Start at the back of your head where you can imagine the two large tendons that connect to the muscles that go across your shoulders. And imagine you are a little searchlight that scans up and down these muscles like a security guard, but there's nothing to see now, and you can relax and take a break. Imagine you lay yourself down on these wide and flat muscles like someone laying down at the top of a grassy knoll, in the sun, on a warm day, under a warm blanket.

Now your lymphatic system is an odd looking thing. It's not big where you're big, and it bears no weight. It's more like the filigree of mushroom mycelium running through the garden bed of your body. It has no nerves, it doesn't bleed, and you can't strain it, so we'll have to talk a little bit about it.

Your body has 6 quarts of blood that circulates through you every twenty seconds. Your body has 1 quart of lymphatic fluid and it takes a day to travel through your body. You wouldn't even know to pay it any attention, and that's just fine. But today we will and it will give us a little tour.

Your blood is pumped through your lungs, throughout your body, and then it returns. Your lymphatic fluid goes only one way, back into your heart. It isn't pumped from anywhere, it just accumulates throughout all your tissues because it leaks from the blood and saturates your tissues like water passing through a sponge.

It is the garbage chute. It is what's washed away from all your cells to be perfectly recycled. Cleaned, examined, restored, and returned to the blood plasma from whence it came.

It is the army barracks, where the soldiers of your body—your white blood cells—while away the time of their short lives—they only live a few days—waiting in case they're needed.

It is the check-point, the outpost, where the signatures of health carried in your fluids are checked, examined, recorded and—when something is amiss—where chemical alarms are sent out and reinforcements called to be released into your bloodstream and directed toward the suspects.

And there is no heart to move your lymphatic fluid, it's all done by other pressures, enhanced by movement and impeded by tension. An active heart moves blood, and an active body moves lymphatic fluid. It is your movement that is the pump, alternately contracting and releasing.

And you must have water—it's fundamental for all processes. You are really a water being. A bag of fluid in a Gore-Tex skin, always losing water so you must constantly replace it. And your immunity requires this, and you will drink enough, you will know because you'll feel moist, you'll pee a lot, and you'll always respond to that dry feeling by reaching for water.

So this is the system we'll travel through. One you've never seen and never will, so you'll have to learn it by heart, by touch, by feel, and by memory. You'll have to invent it like a character in a dream, but, of course, those characters are real, too. They speak the messages to you that your inner self wants you to know. And the characters of your lymphatic system will speak to you also, and you'll build a relationship with them, and they'll speak the messages that your body wants you to know.

So, let's begin.

Relax your brow, and your temples, and relax the bridge of your nose, and the sockets of your eyes, and the hinge of your jaw. Let your jaw drop just a little so that your tongue has some air above it. And settle back beneath your ears to the back of your head where those muscles are, and let them just balance without any stress or strain. Just attached between your skull and shoulders like the hawsers of an old boat moored to a dock on a crystal calm sea.

And as everything is quiet in the territory of your muscles you can rotate your awareness around your neck to the front, and to either side of your trachea, your windpipe, and that delicate area that runs up to beneath your chin from your collarbone, into the soft glands inside and below your jaw, those glands that swell when you get a cold.

Those are our first stations: the glands of your lymphatic system that swell when they become the staging area for military operations in your throat and sinuses. They are not swollen now, or maybe they are, but in either case feel that area now. Focus your attention there and you can imagine, or maybe you can sense, numerous glands with neither muscle nor nerves, that are between the size of peas and almonds, buried in your soft tissues. Pause for a moment. Breath and relax. Remember what this feels like.

Move your awareness down the lines of your neck to your shoulders, to the collarbone's broad lipped plateau running from shoulder joint to shoulder joint. Fixate on your shoulders. Focus in on your shoulder joints, moving your attention around their solid mass to the soft tissue below them, your armpits.

These hollow and sensitive areas which, for some odd reason, are full of nerves—as if tickling is a necessary function. Moving inside your armpits to an area we instinctively protect as vulnerable and sensitive. An area filled with lymph nodes. Nodes that form outposts of protection for our lungs, that add to our fluids and monitor infection in our lungs and thorax.

Take a slow breath. Inhale… and exhale… and fill these areas inside your armpits with a soft energy. Relax the circulation, relax the glands, relax the muscles. Take another breath, inhale… exhale… and imagine these glands filled with the attentive corpuscles, T-cells, and other agents of your defense. Imagine that, like a platoon, they are aware of your effort, and they dispatch a kind of "wave" to let you know they appreciate your attention.

Now, I'd like you to move your hands and lay them over your heart, the hands that you had laid upon your abdomen—place your thumbs on your collarbone, fingers laid over fingers, atop your sternum, resting above your heart.

And this is where you instinctively reach when emotionally startled or overwhelmed. We say we place a hand over our heart, but it's not just our heart we're covering, it's also our thymus gland which nestles just above it.

The thymus is the nursery of your immunity, where your body forms and trains the T-cells critical for your defense. Cells that travel like knights of the realm to patrol our bodies. Like samurai. And this is what lies below the knuckles of your hands. Let yourself sink into this area and look around. What do you see? What do you feel? Relax and imagine your hands are energy, and they can pass through your tissues like ghosts, and they do, and just behind the bone they find the lilac-colored, fatty tissue of your thymus.

Take a breath and let the energy of the breath infuse this area, just between your lungs so that the cool energy of the air mixes with the warm energy of your hands to heat and ventilate this area in your mind, like clean clothes taken from the dryer, to warm your chest. And you will remember what this feels like in the active, bustling avenue beside your aorta.

Now bring your hands down just two inches lower, and slide your right hand leftward to below your left breast, with your left hand atop your solar plexus. Beneath your right hand, within your rib cage, just at the base of your left lung is your spleen, a dark, flattened, purple organ that is another filter for your blood and the central depot of your red and white blood cell reserves.

Focus on this area, an area we hardly notice, and see if you can feel the presence of your spleen. An organ that draws together both circulatory and lymphatic systems, a highway of veins, capillaries, and ducts. The spleen is a dual-function organ both filtering the old lymph and fostering new white blood cells. Both cleaning and nursing in the same organ.

Imagine an energy radiating from the palm of your right hand into the spleen, as if it was a magnifying glass that concentrated the light of the sun, and your spleen was a thick, succulent leaf that absorbed this energy to become more robust. Take a moment to breathe into it. Inhaling into your spleen the oxygen from your lungs, fortifying it like water to young plants. And exhale… to wash away impurities, to be carried off with the energy of your breath. Inhale… and exhale.

Move down the center of your body to your lower abdomen, and let your two hands rotate over each other to slide down and to come to a rest where they started, over your lower stomach. Your fingertips on your pubic bone, your thumbs touching, and your palms over your small intestines.

Antibodies are produced in your small intestines, crucial in fighting infection. A rich supply of lymphatic nodes stores these, blanketing the area to either side of your gut. Direct the energy from your hands into these areas on either side, these peripheral tissues lying between your lower gut and pelvic bones, beneath your palms. Send your positive energy into these nodes, like care packages from home. Relax this area. Use the sides of your hands to press into this area. Press, release, and relax.

Small nodes line this area—without veins or arteries, bones or nerves—forming a network of outposts above the rodeo of your digestion. Press, release, and relax. Just below and beside them are your hip joints, and imagine, now, there is warmth and comfort in this region. Press, release, and relax.

Your palms project warmth and light and imagine that your tissues light up, as if glowing from ultraviolet light emanating from your palms, like fluorescent minerals, centers of energy, storehouses of protection. And in response to this, confirming the message was received, your intestines glow just faintly. Home to trillions of foreign cells living in the folds and lining of your gut, contributing to your health as members of the ecosystem that is you.

Through these areas, and all the others we've visited, run the lymphatic ducts, layered between muscle, passing beside organs, carrying the slow movement of a clear fluid of cellular waste and white blood cells back toward your heart where they'll be debriefed, repaired, replaced, and returned to your blood.

Hovering above, look down on yourself from head to toe. See the glands in your neck nestled behind your bones and in your throat, and the glands buried deep in your chest, in the areas of your armpits, and those fanning left and right above your pelvis. All locations that we move a lot, the arms, neck, and legs. All muscle areas that are messaged when you walk and move.

Your thymus—woven into the highways of your heart and lungs—and your spleen—wedged in between your stomach and your rib cage. This strange system functions as one, collecting and coordinating its many agents and mechanisms. You're vaguely aware of it, like someone who receives sporadic letters from a relative in the secret service. And you can be more attentive to it. Open a channel of communication so that you follow these directions, and you move in ways that contribute to its flow.

You will hear and attend to it. It asks too little of you, so you must motivate yourself, sending packages of energy to these silent troops who are, as yet, unaware of your new willingness to help.

You are above yourself looking down, and inside yourself looking around, and at these locations listening. And you have built ideas and images that you can remember. Pictures and senses of warmth, movement, and relaxation.

Those mysterious bumps and tingles, pops and flashes that occur during the day have meaning, and you'll stop and listen to them. You'll survey them before you go to sleep, like taking a walk through the woods, through the jungle, through the fantastic society of your body and your being.

Relax now. Take a breath. Inhale… exhale… Let yourself float, let your mind wander, let your sensations drift away. Recall only the warm memories, like snapshots of a great trip to a foreign land. A land of unfamiliar features and strange languages.

The pulsing, glowing, translucent landscape that underlies your being and to whom you can now speak a few words, like a tourist carrying your Berlitz book of helpful phrases. You can ask, "How are you?" "Where is the bathroom?" "I need your help." "What do you need?" and "How can I help you?"

And how can I help you? I can help you to relax; to listen to your body. Inhale… exhale… sleep.

4 – Become An Activist

Recognize, declaim, insist, and agitate for what's important.

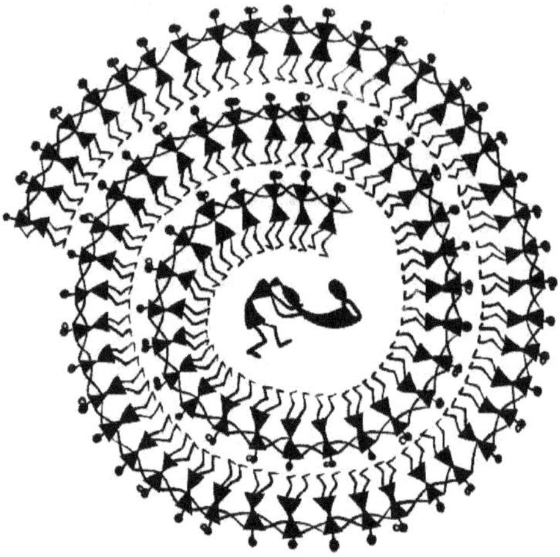

"You must become an activist if you are going to live the natural life."
— **Clarissa Pinkola Estes**

You

As an individual, your family is your constellation. Your primary goals are safety and continuity. Safety means being free from illness, and continuity means being free to grow. Recognize that neither politics, media, nor healthcare share these goals. In fact, they don't even act to further them. They create a context that provides resources for them.

Politics wants your support and, for politicians, the goal is to stay in office. Healthcare wants to fulfill patient needs. Its goal is a smooth operation. The media wants your attention. They're paid to get it.

This is not cynicism, this is how it works, how it balances. And it does balance, more or less, when social forces remain within limits. But they're not within limits now, and you should not be surprised that the system no longer meets your needs.

Truth

Science is hesitant. Politics is partisan. The media are sensational. Healthcare is a service. The virus is dangerous. Add these all together and you get a spectacle of sensational partisan services balanced by scientific hesitancy. There is a danger, but you won't see it clearly by following either the media, the doctors, or the politicians.

The honest media can't tell you the truth because they have to tell a simple story aimed at a middle-school readership. For the most part, the media has been selling a biased, tabloid version of events for so long that they can no longer follow the real evidence. Those journalists who have the skills to explore the truth have moved out of the mainstream.

Honest politicians can't tell you the truth because they're beholden to the social good, and the social good does not address your needs or your knowledge. At best, politicians protect what they see as the center of the flock, leaving the boundaries exposed.

In a crisis, the center of the flock is exposed. It's no longer enough to keep an economic shell intact and social services running when citizens have no income and hospitals can't save people. What's needed is the fostering of mass support for quality, equity, and innovation. This is beyond what the political system is able to deliver.

Health services can't tell you the truth because they see you only as a potential patient. Like distracted parents, they focus only on your safety when you're in crisis. They see only that part of the population that needs what they provide, that part that fits within their care model. For the most part, hospitals are only providing intensive care services, even though your best chance of recovery requires intervention before you need intensive care. Once you require intensive care—the point at which you're on the doctor's radar—your chance of mortality has risen to 20% or higher.

The truth emerges slowly. It's not in any hurry. Those who advocate it do not shout from the rooftops. The truth is not necessarily certain, so don't look to science to declare it. It consists more of clues than conclusions.

As a truth-seeker, you must recognize that different people have different truths: the healthcare worker, the politician, the business owner, the worker, the elder, the college student, the child. Each is impacted differently, and has different goals, obligations, and risks.

There is no one truth that fits all, but there is one truth that no group will inform or announce, and that's your truth. You must be your own detective and come to your own conclusions.

Social Obligation

Your safety is very different from social safety. You know you are not a statistic. As far as institutions are concerned, however, that's all you are. For example, elections, vaccines, and public education are designed to further social goals, not personal ones. They may succeed at one—fortifying society—and fail at the other—thus damaging your family—and still meet the goals for which they are designed.

You want to know how safe you are, not how safe the population is. Knowing that requires a new variable, one you won't see mentioned in the papers, by healthcare professionals, or by politicians—and that variable is your particular situation.

I'll assume you are either in a group that consists of healthy children, youths, parents, workers, and retired elders, or you are in that group of people who have pre-existing illnesses or weakened health. I was surprised to find the relative sizes of these two groups are largely uncertain. Estimates of the size of the healthy group range from anywhere between four times larger than the unhealthy group to the two groups being of equal size. That's a huge uncertainty.

Safety

Two details about COVID-19 that have been misreported or conceals are the means of infection and the percentage of those infected who display symptoms. We have been told to focus on transmission by touching and to fear contagion from those who are showing symptoms. I strongly doubted surface contact was the main mode of transmission or that those showing symptoms were the main threat. Now, four months from these initial warnings the CDC is changing their opinion: "contact transmission," as it's called, is not considered a predominant risk. According to Dr. Robert Redfield of the Centers for Disease Control and Prevention, at least 25% of the people who are transmitting the virus may be asymptomatic (Ghose, 2020).

There is compelling evidence that the virus can be transmitted by inhaling enough of the air recently exhaled by an infected but asymptomatic person. To minimize this possibility, the public has been told to adhere to a "6-foot rule," in which a social distance of at least six feet is maintained between persons at all times. There is no rational for this number; it has simply been pulled out of thin air on the basis that some standard is better than none (Ghose, 2020), and that is certainly true.

When aerosolized, the SARS-CoV-2 virus can remain airborne for hours. Transmission by air remains a central controversy. See Roxanne Khamsi's article, "They Say Coronavirus Isn't Airborne—but It's Definitely Borne By Air".

Wearing a face mask lowers the viral load but does not ensure your safety. Your protection from others—and their protection from you—is not guaranteed. By lowering the viral load you, or they, are slowing the speed and lessening the likelihood of transmission, but not guaranteeing that it won't happen. To guarantee safety, you need both a Hazmat suit and a respirator. But remember, most people with a strong immune system won't get sick even if thoroughly exposed.

The moral of the story is that you must think statistically, to weigh your chances against your risks. I suspect that most healthcare workers who deal with infected patients all day have already been exposed and are already infected. I would presume their continued lack of symptoms indicates that as long as they keep their exposure low, they won't become symptomatic.

Preventing yourself from being an unwitting vector of infection is a different story. Here, we can all act as role models even when we don't know if we're infected, infectious, or immune. By following certain protective conventions—even if it's just a matter of ceremony—we encourage others to do the same. And of those others, there's a good chance that someone who would otherwise be a vector will have that role contained.

The use of face masks is becoming widespread, and will continue to be required more widely. If you've ever used a face mask—to protect yourself from dust or fumes—then you'll know that only a respirator offers guaranteed protection against airborne contagion; see: "Protective Equipment to Healthcare Employees' Skin and Clothing" (Casanova, Alfano-Sobsey, Rutala, Weber, & Sobsey, 2008).

The N95 "respirator" that we hear about is hardly a respirator in real terms; it's hardly effective as such under the front-line multiple-use of donning and doffing, and the persistently contagious conditions we have.

I live in a separated household. My son travels back and forth between me and his mother twice a week. She and I spend little time in each other's presence, but my son is in close contact with us both. In general, we share all illnesses and I'm sure this is the case in most families. In spite of this, we don't all display the same symptoms, even after accounting for the delays in transmission.

In my case, I started running a fever before anyone else in my family. I could have caught the virus from outside, but, whether I caught it from or gave it to him, my son now has it. And from him, his mother has caught it, too. Yet neither of them show any symptoms.

I can't be sure this is COVID-19, but it demonstrates that not everyone who gets a virus shows symptoms. We don't know how contagious asymptomatic people are or if there's a way to distinguish more contagious people from less contagious people, but, given the rapid spread of COVID-19 well before cases started being confirmed, it appears that asymptomatic people are a main means of transmission.

Health

Those with pre-existing illnesses constitute a separate group suffering a mortality rate elevated by a factor of 100. Where COVID-19 can sicken healthy people—and we still don't know how often it does this, although the figure has currently dropped to around 0.5%—it often kills unhealthy people. You may be in the unhealthy group, or someone in your family may be. In that case, you must consider your family, as a group, to be at risk.

Just because COVID-19 is not a significant threat to you doesn't mean it isn't a threat for others. Just because SARS-CoV-2 is not in your area now, and you are safe for the moment, doesn't mean you will continue to be safe. The changing nature of the situation is not being explained by any of the three vocal groups—politicians, media, or healthcare providers. They need your attention and they know that people, in general, won't sacrifice for the public good unless they feel threatened. They're willing to cause you discomfort so that you'll follow their directions.

This has not worked out well for opinion planners; it was a flawed strategy. The stratagem of asking people to make sacrifices for a threat that does not yet exist, on the pretense that it does, can only be carried on for so long. Not surprisingly, people in unaffected areas started to claim the virus was a pretense for a power grab. Others politicized the issue, casting blame on other countries. What people should have been doing was preparing themselves, but since good information was lacking that meant they would have needed to be educating themselves.

It's unclear whether policymakers in the US decided to withhold details of where the virus was and who was at greatest risk, or whether they didn't know. They certainly made no attempt to provide general education or bring people together. Both of these approaches were being taken in other countries—namely Germany and New Zealand—to positive effect. In the US, politicians at all levels ignored the leading health authorities who were adamant about the need for testing, and the federal government dismissed the situation and did nothing. It's fair to say the authorities were unprepared.

If people are acting for the social good without being stampeded to do so, things are under control. While fear is a great motivator—probably the best—it quickly gives way to all manner of poor thinking. Shouting "Fire!" in a crowded theater does not yield many options.

Not being frightened will further your clear-headedness, and that of others. You'll be better able to support your social obligations and you'll be in a better position to learn, communicate, and understand.

Many people have a weak social conscience, which means they'll act from a high degree of self-interest. If you are one of these people, you'll better appreciate why fear is used as a tool for shaping social thought. We are all selfish, to some extent, and it's something we can use to better understand why we should be less selfish.

Fear shuts down options. Removing fear opens the possibility for people to act altruistically, which one can't do when in jeopardy. It is unfortunate that fear sown by unprepared authorities undermines the altruism society needs.

One of the reasons I moved to Canada was to experience what appears to be a higher level of social consciousness. From what I see, this is definitely the case. But this altruism is not so high that all decisions are beyond reproach. Institutional interests, though somewhat fewer than in the US, still dominate the Canadian landscape. The deals made in back rooms may be just as exploitative, but public altruism is high.

I assume you understand that while COVID-19 may not threaten you individually, it may threaten your social and economic context. This is one of those cases where individual and social needs are intertwined. Establishing a connection between these two objectives should be an educational objective. They do seem to try to encourage this in early education in Canada if only by trying to make students feel school is relevant. This is not a priority in US compulsory education programs.

Sickness

There is no cure for COVID-19 yet, which makes me wonder just how hard people are looking. Medical progress is notoriously slow. There is little latitude for experimentation, and no discoveries without it. Doctors and hospitals discover nothing, as that's not what they're there to do. So who is looking?

You might answer, "scientists," but this is not strictly a scientific question. Viral illnesses have been with us much longer than science has been around. There's plenty of what you might call "bush medicine" which is not the same as pseudoscience. As you may know, many of our pharmaceutical "discoveries" come from bush medicine.

Modern medicine has few defenses against viruses, but many against bacteria. We're told the SARS-Cov-2 virus causes the COVID-19 "disease," but COVID-19 is an infection, not a disease, and it appears to come in a wide variety of forms—so many, in fact, that it can lead to many illnesses. We need more "out of the box" thinking.

The 1918 Spanish Flu infected 30% of the world's and killed 3% of the population. That amounted to 50 million deaths worldwide. That percentage today would be 200 million dead. But it turns out it was not the Spanish Flu that killed these people. It's not clear if the Spanish Flu actually killed anybody, because everybody, according to what's now known, suffered separate, bacterial infections. The flu took down our defenses, but it was our reaction to the bacteria that seems to have killed us (Morens, Taubenberger, & Fauci, 2008; Brundage and Shanks, 2008).

And where do the bacteria come from? They live in your nose, and they're living there now! Pneumococcus, staphylococcus, and streptococcus all normally live in your nose, and we can kill them with antibiotics. But they didn't have antibiotics in 1918; penicillin wasn't discovered until 1928.

If you think science is going to save you from COVID-19, then you should be aware that none of the voices you hear speak for science. Neither politicians, the media, nor doctors discover anything. How about we take these people by the scruff of their necks and drag them in the right direction? We don't have time to wait for this to happen by itself. Be an activist. Use your intuition.

I've created *Unwinding the Negative* as a guided visualization to finding a more relaxed and empowered attitude. An affirmation that you have power and that you are safe. Listen to this piece to become grounded and goal-oriented.

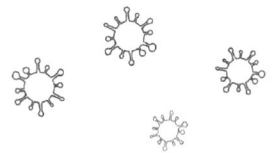

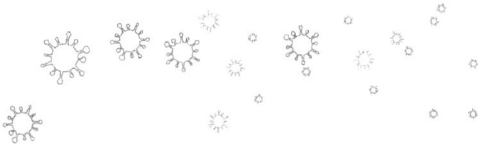

Hypnotic Session 3

Unwinding The Negative audio file at:
https://www.mindstrengthbalance.com/covid19-illness-illumination/

Unwinding The Negative

Unwinding The Negative is a hypnotic induction that requires your full attention. Do not listen to this hypnotic visualization if you are driving a car, operating machinery, or doing anything that requires your attention.

Unwinding The Negative is designed to counterbalance some of the anxiety and the anxiety-producing information that pours into our social awareness. *Unwinding The Negative* doesn't require that you have either skill or experience, it's just a guided visualization, or a guided focus, slow and simple.

Begin this by moving into a calm and relaxed state. It's a state of clear thinking, immune from threats of anxiety, and it provides you with a basis for integrating a grounded sense of being. Being grounded is a state, not a thought; you get there very simply by tuning yourself down, and we can begin that by relaxing your body and calming your mind.

Find a relaxed position: a comfortable chair, relaxing deeply on a couch, or lying on a soft bed. You'll need to be undisturbed, so move to a quiet room and turn off your electronics. Silence your cell phone and put a "Do Not Disturb" sign on your door. Stop this recording if you need to attend to those things, and then come back and start it again once you're ready.

Now you have your space, and it's a space in which you're safe, and it's quiet, and nothing will happen for the next 15 minutes. You're fine, and you're calm, and you're comfortable. Pay attention to your body and check in to where you're holding tension. There will be some places that are tense, like bear traps waiting to be sprung by some surprise. Maybe your back, or your shoulders, or your neck. Disarm these traps. Relax your tension and breathe into these parts of your body.

Take a deep breath, relax… and let yourself sigh into a long exhale. And on this exhale, let the energy of any tense areas release like steam from a covered pot. Do it once more, just in silence. Inhale… and exhale… Keep this slow breath and make it a little deeper when you notice some tension, and make it a little shallower when you want to drift.

Let's take your emotions down a few notches. Let's put your thoughts in a jar. Let's pack your mind with stuffing, like the dentist who puts cotton in your mouth. Let's put some cotton in your ears. Don't worry, we're not doing any drilling, we're just adding pillows, and you can take them out at any time.

Moving into a calm mind is a skill and it takes practice, and you'll get better with practice. The next time you listen to this you'll get further, deeper. This time, you'll go just where you're most comfortable.

We'll count our way down, just by counting numbers. Counting backwards starting at one hundred, and counting down by one, and you can count silently, with me, or out loud. And each number is like a wad of cotton, a pillow, or a beach ball. Or maybe a massage therapist pressing the heel of their hand into the muscles of your back.

Start at **100** and say, "Very relaxed."

Pause to finish your breath, and on the next breath say, "**99**… very relaxed."

Pause… inhale… "**98** very relaxed… **97** very relaxed" and we'll just keep going getting more relaxed.

96 very relaxed… **95** very relaxed… **94** very relaxed.

And let these numbers just satisfy your need to talk to yourself.

93 very relaxed. So that you don't need to think any other thoughts just listen to yourself.

92 very relaxed… **91** very relaxed. And there's no hurry, you're doing it just fine.

90 very relaxed… **89** very relaxed… **88** very relaxed. Let these numbers have some space without thought, just like painted numbers.

87 very relaxed… **86** very relaxed. Let yourself slide into a comfortable emotion more calm than you've been in days.

85 very relaxed… **84** very relaxed. Maybe calmer than you've been in weeks.

83 very relaxed… **82** very relaxed. Just imagine these numbers are a train and we are attached to it.

81 very relaxed… **80** very relaxed. And now we can let that train go, and see it in your mind as it pulls away.

70 very relaxed… **60** very relaxed. And it rattles away into the distance.

50 very relaxed… **40** very relaxed. The sounds are just an echo fading to quiet.

30 very relaxed… **20** very relaxed… **10, 9, 8... 3, 2, 1,** and it's gone.

And that's the part that you can practice, the taking-the-train part. And each time you do it, imagine the train has left you in some different place. Maybe in the woods, somewhere in the prairie, or at a quiet train stop, and just let the train take all your talking off on some holiday where it won't come back for another 15 minutes,

Now you're calm and your mind is quiet, and your emotions are like a still pond. Your emotions influence your thoughts, and if you're in a calm state you'll think calm thoughts.

And now you're more responsive to calm-producing information. Anxiety is still attached to the train, and it will come back later when you need it, so let calm stay with you for a while. The train will circle around, but you've given it the slip, for now—plowing a field of possibilities—and the more calm you have the more you see around you, which makes you more calm and calmer still.

Clear thinking requires calm ground, and we have that, and we can build from here. There has been a lot of information lately and little of it is carefully considered or accurate in what it implies. I'll mention two facts that soften some of the sharp edges so that you can stay more relaxed when that train comes back to get you.

First, there is a general bias known as declinism, which means to decline as in to go down. It means that you're predisposed to negative thinking, and it's not just you it's everyone. This has been bred into us to keep us vigilant. We respond more quickly and respond more clearly to negative things.

The media takes advantage of this by supplying us with a predominance of negative stories, and so does advertising, which is never far behind. And this is normal and you can accept this; it's like a stick, it prods things and makes things move. And you have a thick skin and lots of padding and you can overlook it.

You're shown pictures of agents wearing hazmat suits because you'll pay more attention than if they weren't. You'll be excused for thinking you are in danger but you aren't. It's a picture of danger to make you feel endangered, but you're not, and, actually no one in the picture is going to be infected who isn't already.

The Hazmat suits are not really there to protect anyone in the picture as the agents are up to their necks in contagion and whomever they're helping is already exposed. The suits are a symbol of protection that you're supposed to accept. A rather slim hope of protecting everyone, for which our institutions would like credit. As a protocol to demonstrate some action is better than nothing, and to avoid liability and any accusation of carelessness.

The virus is not a poison gas or radiation that has a known source and a limited extent. The virus is an integral part of the ecosystem. It's now everywhere and it's now estimated that it's been with us like fallen leaves since the middle of January.

I think I've already had my case of COVID-19, it was mild. I live with a family, so they all had it as well, and they showed no symptoms. We isolated ourselves for two weeks, and I think we're now immune. We don't have it and we can't spread it. We've made it to the other side, and you will too. COVID-19 is not a risk to us, and we pose no risk, either.

If you don't have an existing illness, your chances of developing serious complications from this virus are down by a factor of 100. If that's the case for you, then your chances of developing complications are equal to your chances of developing serious complications from the seasonal flu, which is something you've been living with all your life and it hasn't bothered you much. It's the people who have a preexisting illness that are in danger, and those people must isolate, and you must isolate from them. Also, as has been noted, if you're a smoker, now is a great time to quit.

These are the two things to remember: the news emphasizes the negative, and if you're healthy you're in no more danger than you ever were. By holding on to those points we can move back to the center.

Where did the train of numbers leave you? In the woods? In the prairie? At a train station? Wherever you imagine yourself to be, picture it now, in your mind. Picture the woods as if you're in the woods, or the plains if you're in the plains, or the station if you're in the station. And turn around in a circle in your mind and see that it's woods all around, or plains all around, or the station platform runs from side to side.

And in the woods, or in the plains, or in the station there is a post, a signpost. And on it is a golden, yellow, circle with a black outline and black letters, and the sign says, "I DON'T BUY IT." And it means all that negative information, all the warnings of doom and the threats of destruction. And you don't buy it because you prefer, and you respond to, and you act to make happen what you want to see happen. And you have that power, and you can do that.

You approach this sign, and as you do the post gets larger but the sign stays the same size until, when you're right beside it, it's no larger than a gold coin. And you reach up and you take it in your hand and you put it in your pocket, in your bag, or—even better—in your heart. Just like that, you put it in your heart. So now you don't have to think about it because you feel it.

And now you look down at your hands, and you see you're holding a train ticket, an old fashioned blue paper ticket that comes off a roll. The ticket has just one world and that one word is "SAFE." And it means that for the ticket holder—which is you—the virus is done and you are safe. It's over. You've had it and you've recovered, or you have it and you're recovering, or you will have it and you'll recover. This ticket is your certification that it's done, and you're safe.

Of course, it's just a ticket, and there's always the possibility that reservations are overbooked, but that's never a real problem. You should never worry about travel arrangements. So you put this ticket in your pocket, or your bag, or—better yet—in your heart so that you won't forget it.

We'll all get this ticket. I've got mine and now you've got yours. And we'll all get this virus sooner or later, and I'm glad I got it sooner. And if you're at risk, then you'll bite the bullet and you'll wait for this train to pass, and you'll get on the next one where they'll have more services and they'll be able to attend to you.

So now you'll remember; and it's not such a circus. And if you're already immune, then you can come out and help others by distributing food, or stocking shelves, or keeping the system running.

Quiet now. Listen into the silence and you can hear the train coming back. One, two, three, and there it appears, a small dot at the end of the vanishing tracks running from the distance beyond the woods, across the prairie, to the train station. You can see its movement, counting its way toward you: **8**, **10**, **15**, **23**.

And you take a breath, you inhale… and exhale… And relax into your imagination, and you pad your pockets, secure your bag, inflate your chest. And everything is intact as the train rounds the corner, past the last trees, the windswept grasses.

38—hushing to a stop—**39**. The door slides open. You get in, pass the vestibule and go into the cabin. There are rows of seats filled with families returning, and there are kids playing, and dogs in carriers, and suitcases on the racks.

There's an empty seat or an empty row, and if you're alone you take the seat, and if you're with your family you take the whole row. And everyone is comfortable, and the seat is comfortable. The sky is overcast but the weather is good.

The train begins to move; **40**, **41**, **42**, **43**. And you lean your head back, and you close your eyes as the tracks click-clack, the rolling numbers; **49**, **51**, **55**.

As you get yourself up to speed, and you find yourself coming back, counting up. Counting up, back to where you started: **60**, **70**, **80**.

You're calm again, you're comfortable and you're pleased. You've done well and you're confident. It's amazing, and it will be more amazing. And you don't know whether the virus is a curse or a blessing. And it's microscopic and it has no brain, but it has a purpose and it's been at its task for three billion years, and it's got an intelligence that we'll never fathom.

94, **95**, inhale… exhale… **97**, **98**, **99**. And we're back. **100**.

---

5 – Lungs

Hypnotizing your immune system might prevent it from filling your lungs with liquid.

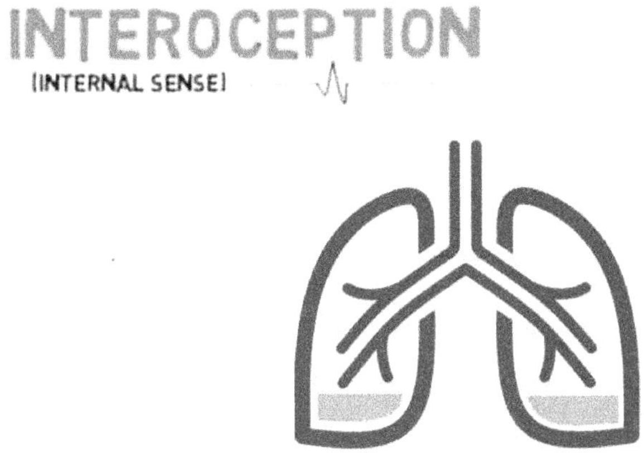

"It is a common belief that we breathe with our lungs alone, but in point of fact, the work of breathing is done by the whole body."
— **Alexander Lowen**, from *The Voice of the Body*.

Totalitarianism

The pandemic crisis has handed governments sweeping, authoritarian powers because people need governments to coordinate economic, social, and medical services. This will amplify the character of governments: good governments will get better, bad ones will get worse, bi-partisan governments will become more collaborative, and sectarian ones more combative. There will be good decisions, bad decisions, heroes, and villains. There will be plenty to be thankful for and plenty of corruption. As is usually the case, the time to make this better was long ago.

The pandemic has also handed the medical establishment total healthcare powers, mostly because they have authority, power, and money. This is not due to their having all the answers or sufficient resources —they have no answers and they don't have enough resources! Let's look at just a few issues with the objective of getting to the topic of hypnosis.

Healthcare authorities advocate testing for reasons of epidemic management and monitoring. This does not tell people what to do or inform them of how serious the threat is. They have been told what to do: isolate; and they know how serious the threat is, as that's measured by mortality, not infection. You don't need to test dead people.

Testing enables authorities to demonstrate to the population and to politicians that they should do what they should already know they should do. Testing is not a strategy against infection, it's a measurement of the situation that provides an argument for an effective response. Testing provides ammunition against foolishness. In a population of the foolish, foolishness is the first means of infection.

Healthcare authorities have been, not been, and sometimes been advocating social distancing, quarantining, shelter-in-place, disinfecting, avoiding touching oneself or others, cloaking, masking, and covering because—we've been told—the virus is transmitted by touch, droplets, and air and can live on surfaces for days. This has been a confusing quagmire of contradictory, inconsistent, unproven, and misleading information. "Keep six feet apart," we're told. A distance for which there is no basis in fact. Ten feet is a better idea.

The only logical connection between the mode of transmission and these suggested measures is keeping people separated. Shelter-in-place appears to be the only measure that has bent the curve of the population's rate of transmission. By themselves, masking, covering, cloaking, washing, and disinfecting did next to nothing on a large scale. These measures don't work unless they're flawlessly put into effect. On the other hand, ceremony is important. It's a form of affirmation and communication. In a culture where faces carry so much meaning, wearing a mask is a huge symbol of consideration and support.

Today I stood in a line of 60 people, properly separated. I would have waited 40 minutes breathing everyone else's air and moisture if I hadn't been disgusted by the farce of it all. I returned my groceries and left the store. Social distancing allows too much "leakage."

On the small scale of individual protection, a full armamentarium of germ isolation can protect the few medical professionals able to maintain it. This Hazmat-suited level of protection is unavailable to the rest of us. It's increasingly unavailable to the frontline providers, too.

Sick-Care Is Not Coming to the Rescue

What do the healthcare authorities have to offer us? They haven't been able to test for COVID-19, they can't stop it, and they can't cure it. Also, if you've been reading carefully, they can't diagnose it symptomatically, as COVID-19 is not only respiratory but also gastrointestinal, and can present as skin rashes, heart attacks, strokes, and organ failures.

Why are we following directions from our doctors, clinics, and emergency providers like children being led by the pied piper? Lemmings would be a better description. Why are we following this medical guesswork so slavishly? You might answer, "Because in the more severe cases they can save my life!" But can they?

Doctors are asked to deny tests to those without symptoms. Hospitals turn away all but the most seriously ill, of whom 20% will require intensive care. Treatment is a combination of poor home care and experimental medicine. Half of those that need a respirator expire. Just like the time to fix the political system is before it falls apart, the best time to secure your health is before you lose it.

I am not impugning the medical system. They're doing exactly what they said they'd do, and they're doing it as best they can. I am chiding the foolishness of relying on them for healthcare. They are an emergency, sick-care system and, if you're not yet sick, then you would do better if you made plans not to get sick or—in the event that you do get sick—not to get so sick.

In Chapter Three, I endorsed measures to boost your immune system. Here, I want to address the issue of survival, which is more about strength than immunity. If immunity is tantamount to how to avoid a sinking ship, then survival is about what to do when it sinks.

Dying

How are you most likely to die from COVID-19? It seems to result from one complication or another having to do with a failure of your cardio-pulmonary system. Either you can't respire and drown outright, or you exhaust your energy and die trying. The respirators might save you if you're exhausted, but they can't help you if your lungs have failed. Might there possibly be some other way of approaching this endgame?

First of all, people don't just drown because they sink. They sink because they can't swim, so staying afloat is your first means of protection. Respirators are breathing tubes for sinking people. How about throwing drowning people a life preserver? What would that mean?

Scuba diving is a sport whose first rule is to not drown. It relies on two primary skills: swimming and breathing. The first involves muscles and the second lung power. Both of these are quickly learned.

If you've ever exercised, you'll know that you become sore and, in a couple of days, you get stronger. Amazing, isn't it? If you've ever done any diving—granted, most people have not, but if you had—you'd know that you can quickly expand your lung capacity. A good scuba diver will use only half the air of an unskilled diver, and they execute the same maneuvers. Part of that is because they use their muscles less, but part of it is also because their respiration is more efficient. Their lungs work better.

Now, I'm going to make what will seem like an outrageous suggestion for everyone: get serious exercise now, and exercise your breathing! Spend an hour each day getting cardio-pulmonary exercise. Can you imagine the uproar that would ensue if the government required this? Imagine being forced to learn to survive! What an unprecedented invasion of privacy! Would it be too much to expect this be recommended?

Hypnotism

Being calm lies at the root of not drowning. First, the reason you have liquid in your lungs is that your immune response has gone haywire, it has created the liquid that is drowning you. If you know anything about the behavior of a drowning person, you will know that they effectively doom themselves by not knowing what to do, and by exhausting themselves doing the wrong things, which is not unlike your immune system. If you could hypnotize a drowning person to cease their panic they wouldn't drown, they'd float.

I'm going to make another outrageous suggestion—more outrageous than the last one—which is that by hypnotizing your immune system to relax, it might not fill your lungs with liquid. You can say that's ridiculous, and it might be, but hypnotism does some amazing things because people can do some amazing things, a lot more than they're told they can do. Gaining some control over one's immune system is well within the limits of what's possible.

If we expect 30% of the world's population to contract COVID-19 and 1% of those to die—which is optimistic—then 20 million will die. If hypnosis could relax the immune reaction and save 1% of these, 200,000 who would otherwise die, would live. The effect could actually be ten times that number, and, in addition, survivors would get better faster.

There's another benefit: a relaxed person needs less air. This is half of the magic of a successful diver: you learn to exert almost no force when swimming as all your unused muscles are limp. A drowning COVID-19 patient is going to be struggling. They're afraid and they're gasping for air. Struggling is not helping, but it only seems rational.

Hypnosis isn't rational. You can sweep away any level of pain, and separate yourself from any reality. It is actually quite easy to hypnotize a person into a level of deep relaxation, and in this state, your muscles will not consume much oxygen or produce much CO2.

I don't know how much pressure this would take off your strained cardio-respiratory system, but it could have some significance. What if it lowered your respiratory requirement by 10%? Would that mean that 10% of those who would otherwise suffocate would survive?

Airways

These are my two suggestions for seriously ill, COVID-19 patients: relax the immune response, and relax the body's need for air. Toward this end, I've written the hypnotic induction *Airways*.

Airways is written to be an aid for people experiencing pulmonary distress: anticipated, incipient, progressing, serious, or severe. Its goal is to fortify, synchronize, energize, support, and relax all three: the person, the lymphatic system, and the autonomic nervous system. I believe it could save lives.

Hypnotic Session 4

Airways audio file at: https://www.mindstrengthbalance.com/covid19-illness-illumination/

Airways

Airways is a hypnotic induction that requires your full attention. Do not listen to this hypnotic visualization if you are driving a car, operating machinery, or doing anything that requires your attention.

The goal of *Airways* is to relax the immune response in your trachea, bronchial tubes, bronchioles, and pulmonary tissues. It speaks to your listening mind, but addresses the muscles, cilia, alveolar tissues, lining, and the lymphatic system that controls your pulmonary immune response. It speaks to the tissues in your body. It aims to assist these tissues in relaxing their histamine production, inflammatory reaction, relieve consolidation, and coordinate their response to bronchitis, asthma, emphysema, viral and bacterial pneumonia, and other infections.

We begin here, first by letting gravity sink you down into whatever you're lying or sitting on. Lie back, rest your head and neck. It's important to let your spine relax, so you don't need to stay upright. You want the muscles of your back relaxed because they hold and guide your lungs, and we want your lungs relaxed and also aware and in control. Your spine is the trainer wheels, a crib's railing to your body's organs and we want to let your lungs have all the control to speak and see and explore.

If you're breathing is troubled, breathe with your body. Feel your body expand on the inhale and relax on the exhale, your lungs only moving as much as is comfortable. With each exhale imagine the breath exiting the top of your head, steam exiting the rim of a lidded pot, so with each breath you're more relaxed and your mind more empty.

The air you're exhaling slips under the lid of the pot at the top of your head, so all the thoughts of your mind juter past like scraps sliding off a dustpan. Sweep them up, and shake them out… up and out… counting down.

Inhale lightly, **ten**, deeply relaxed… exhale...

Inhale lightly, **nine**, deeply relaxed… exhale...

Inhale, **eight**, and the more you relax the better it feels.

Seven, inhale, deeply relaxed… and exhale...

Inhale, **six**, deeply relaxed… exhale...

Five, deeply relaxed. Sinking deeper into the warmth of your body.

Four, deeply relaxed. Calm, limp, and released.

Three, deeply relaxed down to the roots of your teeth and the edge of your awareness.

Two, deeply relaxed. Breathing calmly and without effort.

Down to **one**, to the beginning of our voyage… into your body, into your cells. Into the microscopic world of chemical messages, molecules, markers juggling meanings.

Imagine you can sense the movement of air through your body, as if you could see into yourself as you breathe. You have the eyes of air that swales past your nostrils and drops down your throat like a well. And on this course, you pass your tongue and larynx, down your esophagus to a sharp turn past the stern and never-failing epiglottis, gate into your trachea where the landscape changes to a fluted air-like passage, a softer and more motile surface conveying a thin film of clear and liquid mucus always upward on the upside-down feet of a million cilia, always pedaling it out, because that's all they ever do, and what makes their life complete.

You are traveling with the air, and the air is more than just a vehicle like the water carrying a boat in the sea. The air, like the sea, is a life-giving substance, not living in itself but a carrier of life, like the plasma in your blood which carries salts and proteins. The air carries oxygen and carbon dioxide. And, you know, these are mysterious elements that you cannot judge as simply good or bad. They can be poisonous, just as too much salt or sugar is poisonous, but they are essential in their balance because it's only in balance that your system lives and moves, so you must always reach out to them.

Imagine the smell and taste of fresh air, mountain air, air after a rainstorm or a thunderstorm, or ocean air, or forest air. This is oxygenated air and it is restorative. All air you breathe has oxygen available to you.

As you follow this air into your lungs imagine it is perfused with oxygen, a clear gas with a dry taste and a satisfying smell. And as this gas moves deeper into your lungs the blood that moves close to the surface of your tissues attracts it like iron filings to a magnet, and it is much like this but in reverse. It is the oxygen that is the magnet and the blood that is the iron and the blood rusts red as the cells pull oxygen through the tissue thin walls.

And the carbon dioxide that has been carried in your blood is now an acid, carbolic acid, and when it enters your lungs it's neutralized and forms gas again, and it escapes.

Relax the muscles in your lungs. There are muscles like rubber bands wound around your bronchials like bands around matches, or kindling, or packages of spaghetti, and you want to be able to make these tighter or looser as you know they need to be. Sometimes they're too tight and there's too much constriction, more than necessary. It can be overdone.

Imagine that constriction now. And it's not just one handful of muscles, and it's not just one passageway, but many descending downward from your esophagus. These passages split and split again, like cauliflower, branching out at right angles, and each branch has its own muscles toning and tightening the diameter of these ever-multiplying tubes. You can imagine them tightening and constricting and closing down, and you can feel the tightness this creates, and the shallowness of the air.

And next, without stopping to let the tensions set, release these tensions and let all of these open and their muscle-bound rings release, slip, flatten, fatten, and expand as a multitude of small passages open. And leave them open for the airing, so that as you inhale your diaphragm opens the passages, as if you're opening the barn doors of a garden shed to let the sun in and the moisture out...

Pay attention to the scope and range of your breath. You will notice there is always something that blocks your inhale when your lungs are full. Usually, at the same time as you have a sated feeling, as if you've swallowed just enough. But resistance can also come before you feel you've inhaled enough.

Imagine being very thirsty but only being able to drink in little sips. You may not have this feeling now, or you might, or you might be able to imagine it. If you can't feel it, then make it up. Take small breaths and imagine that is all the air you could take in, or that is how you felt when you took in all the air you could. Explore this feeling without judgment or pressure. Don't strain, relax.

I'm asking you to imagine what might otherwise seem like a suffocating feeling, but not to react to it that way. Recognize that you can recalibrate yourself to need less air. You can relax your body so that your metabolism slows down. Deeply relaxed as when you're in a deep sleep.

If you can do this, then your immune system may relax, too. You'll feel more comfortable and you'll be able to focus in more detail on the sense of limit or resistance. Maybe there is a pain, or maybe there just seems to be no more space. Imagine you can soothe it, contain it, and make it smaller. If it's a resistance or block, then imagine you can put a different pressure on it, or get some kind of message about its nature so that you can better work with it, to massage or relax it.

You will only be breathing with the muscles that you know, and when there is resistance it's natural you will try harder, breathing in the same way. Explore your hundreds of muscles to see how else you might breathe. Can you breathe with different movements in your ribs, or diaphragm? Can you imagine different parts of your diaphragm moving, perhaps breathing more from one side or the other, or from your stomach? Can you imagine breathing from one nostril or the other?

Become aware of your pulse as you breathe. If you have been straining, then you will hear your pulse in your ears. If you are relaxed, then you will feel your pulse as a rhythmic presence inside you, not a sensation or a sound, but a distraction. It will be in your mind, it will force pauses in your train of thought. Your heart beats in the spaces between your silently thought ideas and spoken sentences. Start to dance with this: the thoughts, the breath, the pauses. Coordinate, focus, and synchronize.

See, sense, hear, think, or imagine that your heart beats a little faster and a little stronger, a little harder when you inhale. Stretch out your inhales across several beats even if you have to make them slow and shallow. And at the end of each inhale let your heart beat once or twice and feel it settling down, calming to a relaxed state.

Imagine on your inhale that your heart beats with a vigor as if it was churning butter, pushing against a paste. And at the end of your breath this pressure stops and with your exhale your heart becomes a baker lazily folding dough, stretching and folding once with each beat.

This effort moves back and forth, from butter churning to dough folding as you inhale, pause, and exhale. And you can do this no matter how deep or shallow your breathing, and you'll find it helps your breathing because it's what your heart and lungs know to do. It's a cooperation, like skipping rope or pushing a swing, and the two work together and your whole system falls into an even pace.

This ability to synchronize is called heart rate variability. It will make your breathing easier. It's well known, important, and it correlates with your inflammatory response. Your body can learn to do this quickly. There are many ways to learn it, but I think this is the easiest: listening to your heart. And this is so important here, when your lungs are under threat.

Your heart is your lungs' partner and you must work with it. Your lungs are the eyes of your heart in the same way that your eyes are the windows of your soul. Where your eyes see, your lungs sense.

Your lungs are a skin, an internal skin that has its own surface layer. It has a much bigger surface than your external skin, thirty times larger: the area of a tennis court. It is your lungs that are in real contact with the outside, not your skin, it's just that your lungs aren't blanketed with nerves so that you can't feel the contact. The contact is chemical not mechanical.

Realize how big your lungs are so that you understand why you must now pay such close attention. Survey them in detail and you can only see all parts of your lungs from far above. Develop new communications as you have no eyes to see or fingers to touch the surfaces and passages of your lungs. You must think chemically, biologically, and electrically.

You want to address, speak to, show concern for, heal, and protect every inch of your lungs' surface. You want to speak to a very thin layer of liquid blood spread in a microscopic thinness over this huge tissue surface. Where your blood is hidden well beneath your outer skin, it is only separated by a thin membrane here.

Here in your lungs, every blood cell participates. Your lungs are the viewing platform for your blood to see the world, and you must speak to each cell, which is active and present here.

Most of the cells are your red blood cells, and they are not too interested in what you have to say. They are quite single-minded as their chemical interests are narrow and occupied: pull in the oxygen, catalyze the carbolic acid, exhale the CO2, and when finished, move out of the lung and back into the body. Their time in the lung is short, only a few seconds, and their life is months long.

They know what to do and how to do it, and all they need is to make contact and move on. You want to speak to the tissues of your lungs to expedite your red blood cells' passage, make them comfortable, give them the short time of contact they need and move on. Become aware of those areas in your lungs that are granting free passage and those areas that are not. Broadcast this information, like traffic radio, to the red cells in your blood.

The white blood cells are really the victims and the culprits in pulmonary dysfunction. They are a small group by number, only 1% of your blood, but they are active, alive, and individual. They each make their own decisions and their lifetimes are measured in hours. For them nothing is preordained, they are always looking, always curious, and rather headlong and impetuous in their behavior. They come in many shapes with different structures and requirements. The most numerous are the neutrophils, born in your bone marrow and small enough to leak into their outside world inside your lungs. And they will do that, like dogs chasing cars, if you don't train them not to.

When they sense infection, they will leak into your alveolar chambers and they will fill those chambers with pus, and that is what's called consolidation and hardens your lungs and causes your breath to fail.

Tell them not to chase after cars that are the bacteria, viruses and whatever pathogen they smell. Let them stay in the bloodstream because your breathing is more important. They should wait for instructions and let them communicate those instructions among themselves.

In doing this you are preventing liquid from accumulating where it should not. You are preventing pneumonia. There will be those neutrophils who cannot help themselves, and there should be some, and they will form some liquid in your lungs.

You want to expel that liquid, have the cilia lining of your lungs move that liquid up and out. Cough it out, spit it out, or swallow it. You have a conveyor system to clear your lungs, and you should use it. Like a wind sweeping across a lake's surface, your lung's membrane carries this liquid out to clear up congestion. Drying, clearing, and cleaning.

Relax your chest. Let your chest rest imagining all the scouting and trailing, posting and broadcasting you've been doing. Imagine all the millions of minions you've instructed, each with their own family and future, each playing a role and keeping your system in balance.

Deepen your breath as is comfortable. Let your chest move, spreading the movement across all the tissues and throughout your rib cage. Make sure that every inhale expands comfortably in all comfortable directions.

Follow the exhales out; follow all the bronchioles, a net of growing branches spreading over the whole tennis court of your lungs, all neatly folded and spun into two lobes no larger than your chest. With every inhale this quart of air is neatly run across three thousand square feet, and with every exhale it's all recollected and ushered out.

Imagine all parts of your lungs used and working to their greatest degree. You're comfortable as your lungs fully expand and contract. With each contraction moisture and liquid are pushed back out, out through the air you breathe and pushed up through the network of tubes, tunnels, and passageways of your lungs.

You're coming back to the sensory and visual world, emerging from the concepts and chemical signals of your heart-lung. Back to the sense of gravity on your bones, and textures on your skin.

Counting from one to ten, moving up your spine.

One, starting in your gut, the deepest place of breathing.

Two, up your ribs to your heart at the center of your chest and lungs.

Three, up to your collarbone, atop your lungs where your airstreams combine.

Four, into your esophagus where air and liquids pass.

Five, up past the humming of your vocal cords.

Six, into the back of your palate, the pharynx where breath, voice, and food intermix.

Seven, into your sinuses for smells and tastes and blowing your nose.

Eight, out your mouth and nose, past your lips and nostrils and into the world.

Nine, you are much calmer now as your heart and lungs are working together.

Ten, reconnecting your outside eyes, and ears, and sense of sound, and sight, and touch.

Feeling relaxed, feeling strong, and confident in health and healing. Allowing your body to work in collaboration, in touch with itself.

---

6 – Stomach

Get beyond the notion that your stomach is there to serve your needs. It's the other way 'round.

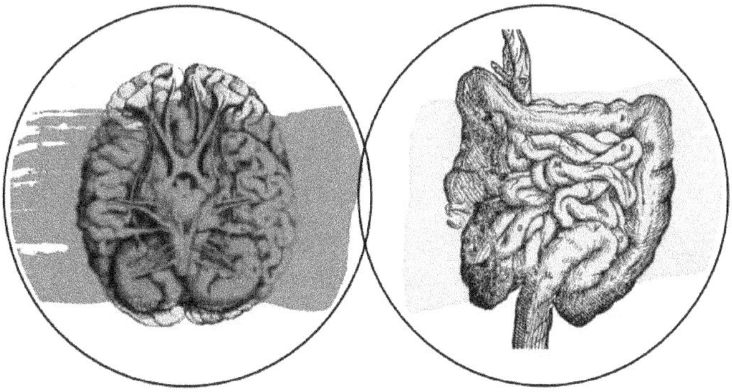

"If your stomach disputes you, lie down and pacify it with cool thoughts."
— **Satchel Paige**

The Gut-Brain Axis

To develop a relationship with your stomach, get beyond the notion that your stomach is there to serve your needs. It's the other way 'round. There are quite a few situations where your stomach is in disagreement with what you want to ingest. Stomach comfort is about what makes your stomach comfortable, which may be uncomfortable from your point of view.

I have a sensitive stomach, but I can't tell whether this means my stomach is reactive or aggressive. My experience has led me to feel that my stomach has a mind of its own and is somewhat fed up with my eating habits. As a result, I now contemplatively consult my stomach before I eat anything.

I recently ate at a nouveau-Mexican restaurant that mixed corn, cheese, hot sauce, whipped cream, bananas, and caramel. My taste buds—which have a short memory—were able to navigate the hairpin curve from pepper-hot to dairy-sweet, but the whole mess didn't go down well. Most of it never made it out of the restaurant.

When you're healthy and hungry, your stomach knows its business and will do yeoman's work to start digestion. But when your health is weak or your stomach disoriented, you need a more mature, mind-stomach relationship. I've never heard anyone else talk about one's mind-stomach relationship, but mine started as a result of my ayahuasca experiences.

To the Jungle, and Beyond!

Ayahuasca is a medicine, ceremony, and other-worldly adventure. Many cultures have herbal knowledge that includes medicinal and therapeutic plant use; of these, ayahuasca is an unusual example. Widely used by Amazonian cultures, ayahuasca is a water-based extraction of a combination of tropical plants whose chemical effect only manifests in combination. The plant constituents are not edible, and the result is so far from palatable that it goes right off the scale.

If you're interested, I have discovered how to simulate the famous taste of ayahuasca: steam a full pound of spinach to get two cups of strangely unappealing, green water. Boil this down to ¼ cup of thick, bitter liquid, mix in a tablespoon of lemon juice, a good pinch of salt, and drink it. I don't think it will hurt you, but I'm sure it will start an unusual experience—an experience which, along with the ideas I'm presenting here, could forever change your relationship with your stomach.

Ayahuasca's traditional mixture combines three ingredients: a dry pound of two tropical plants and the juice of a lemon. If you're short on lemons, use muriatic acid, which we use to scrub pools; it leaves less of a taste. One of the two traditional plants is Psychotria viridis, a shrub in the coffee family. You use the leaves, not the berries. One of Psychotria's relatives, Psychotria emetica, is also called "false ipecac." Ipecac is used to induce vomiting.

The second ingredient, Banisteriopsis, is known as "the vine of the dead." It's a fast-growing, friendly vine whose thick woody stem is beaten to shreds before being added to the pot. The plants and acid are simmered together for many hours. The acid is neutralized to a salty taste. The residue is then strained off and the remaining liquid is boiled down to a black, viscous slurry.

The result is a chemical curiosity of which your stomach will have its own opinion. The experience is entirely different from anything taught in a textbook. Most discussions of ayahuasca center on your head and what happens in your mind, but my focus is on your stomach, and what this experience taught me about mine.

The gastric experience is a cleansing pressure wash, more thorough than any fast or enema. The shamans say the ayahuasca draws toxins from your body which are expelled from your lungs, sinuses, mouth, and anus. The stomach plays a role, but only one of several.

Among ayahuasca's many mental effects is mild anesthesia, somewhat like nitrous oxide, so your senses are muted. In addition, you become highly sensitive to sound, light, and motion; your observations are distorted. The mind-body connection is stretched to the point where it's difficult to walk, having waves of nausea similar to being seasick.

These are just the gross effects. Those who partake in the ayahuasca ceremony always find this joke funny: "How many times do you take ayahuasca for fun? Once!"

It is my habit to prepare for ayahuasca with a day of light eating followed by a two-day juice fast, plenty of liquids and gentle laxatives, similar to how one prepares for a colonoscopy. As a result, when I take ayahuasca it pours down a clear drain. One would expect it to pass right through and, to a large extent, it does.

In the course of many ayahuasca experiences, I noticed something strange. I usually experience secondary nausea ten hours after first drinking the mixture. This secondary nausea generally occurs four to six hours after several waves of expelling from either end followed by hours of sleep and rest. The morning nausea is relieved by vomiting a small amount of liquid. After this, my whole system becomes calm.

The mystery is that the morning vomit appears to be ayahuasca. Judging by the smell and color, what I expel appears to be one of the two distinct plant components that were ingested as a mixture. Hours after first receiving and supposedly passing this medicinal combination, my stomach not only retained but also chemically separated some of the ayahuasca, preventing parts of it from passing through my system.

Everything I've been told about the stomach explains that it serves as an agitator to mix ingested material with gastric fluids which it releases in pulses through the pyloric sphincter into the upper small intestines. This is an incomplete description. My stomach is also sensing, titrating, and unmixing the concoction. It is doing something more sophisticated than simple homogenization.

Incomplete emptying of the stomach is referred to as gastroparesis, and it's recognized as a disability. While there is a lot of "frothy" talk about enteric intelligence, I haven't found any research that identifies what this intelligence does.

It's noted that most of your serotonin and a substantial portion of the body's dopamine is produced in the intestines. 90% of the signals along the vagus nerve are communications from the G.I. tract to the brain. I read comments about mood alteration and emotional intuition that remind me of social talk about racism, where everyone has something to say but no one recognizes it.

What if the stomach intelligence decides what, when, and how much material to release into the intestines? What if this does not constitute a dysfunction, but a considering and proactive stomach? That would mean that many of the mechanical interventions—pharmaceutical, laparoscopic, and surgical—are misguided. It would not be the first time.

What is clear from reading the academic literature is how little we know about the function of the G.I. tract or the role of the enteric nervous system. The G.I. tract shepherds half of the cells in the body and these cells are not human, they are bacteria, fungi, as well as viruses. They are not created in our bodies and do not share human history or DNA. These organisms operate and reproduce on their own.

Communion and Communication

The independent intelligence of my stomach was further clarified to me through a conversation I had with an impatient, old crone who claimed to be my stomach. This voice spoke at a point in one of my hallucinogenic ayahuasca experiences. It was an entirely rational voice that had a brief and succinct message which I have since taken to heart.

I consider hallucinations to be much like trance visions: the experiences are real but their interpretations must be indirect. Like all ideas, hallucinations come from somewhere and represent something. These experiences convey complex structures and meanings that can be vague, concise, emotional, or conceptual. They have all the makings of inspiration in an uncertain context.

Sometimes—though rarely—these hallucinations are verbal, musical, or mathematical. In this case, my hallucination was verbal but, aside from its dissociated origin as the voice of my stomach, it sounded exactly like my own voice.

My stomach told me this: "You don't pay enough attention to what I'm doing, and you eat things thoughtlessly. I get impatient with your insensitivity and I'm not going to make up for your unawareness." I attempted to ask what I should do and whether I could get more direction. The communication channel was already dissolving, but I got the impression that further directions would be available if I looked for them.

That was the last clearly spoken message I heard from her, but it gave me the lasting impression that I should attend, inquire, imagine, and intuit the needs of my stomach and the consequences of my actions. In addition, this brief conversation left me with a certain trust that some force more capable and aware than I was dealing with my gastrointestinal affairs. This has enabled me to approach my own episodes of illness, dysfunction, or discomfort with greater calm and detachment. I now see my mind and senses as playing a more supporting role, and I allow my verbally silent body to coordinate most operations.

Most of our G.I. functions are taboo. The display of its operations is considered socially unacceptable, and this disrespect directly influences our relationship with ourselves. We could psychoanalyze each of our G.I. functions in the manner of Sigmund Freud and benefit from it. I suspect that each of us has personal issues, and these issues offer a direct route to a better understanding of our body. I'll focus on two issues that pertain to my stomach: vomiting and ingestion.

To Vomit or Not to Vomit

Ayahuasca has trained me to be a skilled vomiter. Before ayahuasca, my approach to vomiting was probably the same as yours: painful, repugnant, and depressing. I now recognize these feelings as irresponsible, immature, and unhelpful.

If vomiting is something your stomach needs, then your responsibility is that of an emergency responder. Imagine an emergency responder whose attitude about attending someone in distress is to consider the experience painful, repugnant, and depressing. The only appropriate response one can have to an emergency responder that has that attitude is to punch them.

I have now learned to relax and facilitate vomiting. I have learned to work with my stomach, to calm, endorse, and reassure it. To tell my stomach that I understand its need. I organize my esophagus, breath, tongue, diaphragm, and abdominal muscles to make vomiting painless and efficient.

I have found that, much like any other pain, the painful sensations are due to stress, tension, and expectation. I can remove these forces, and when I do, the discomfort of vomiting is greatly reduced.

I no longer heave, cramp, curse, and sputter like some unpleasant emergency room nurse. Vomiting is now a brief episode of connection, coordination, and relief. My stomach relaxes quickly and I support it entirely. The experience of vomiting is now one of relief.

My stomach does not speak to me in words, but I speak to it, or to her, if I want to anthropomorphize the connection. That's not really necessary. Your stomach has intelligence, and lives in a world you'll never understand. Or will you? I'll leave that for you to determine.

Everything We Eat

You make two decisions before you eat something: is it familiar, and does it taste good. Familiarity is recalled from memory and taste from your tongue. Both of these are imperfect, and neither should be relied upon without consulting your intuition. Many of our eating indiscretions stem from failing to make the wiser choice. But what is intuition?

Intuition is what arises from your subconscious associations and unconscious reflexes. It's information that comes from outside your awareness. The huge range of possibilities is a problem. If you can't judge intuition, then you can't distinguish between good, bad, and indifferent ideas.

Judging intuition is a process that requires sensitivity and attention, similar to channeling spirit, or channeling whatever. It begins with guesswork, memory, and imagination. These create an expectation of where to look and what to see and—once you focus your attention in this manner—something will appear. It's a process of trial and error. The ideas you engage will have some effect in guiding your actions. By judging their effect you improve your intuition.

Eating should not be impulsive, as my Mexican restaurant experience illustrated. The least you can do is to stop and think about it, and when you do you should listen. But listen to more than your memory and your taste buds. Listen to your stomach. Your stomach knows.

Your stomach speaks in inclinations, moods, and reflections, second thoughts and fleeting images. Learn to amplify and retain these, to take them seriously and give them a vote that's equal to your chattering mind and impulsive tastes.

Sugar is a great example. Our taste buds have been programmed to like it, and our memories of sweet things are good. But if you consult your stomach, it will not endorse sugar. Your stomach knows sweet things are a deception like bright flowers to a bee. Sugar wants you to eat it because the candida fungus in your gut thrives on it and candida hijacks your brain.

If you consult the science, you'll find little support for sugar. High fructose diets are associated with both obesity and Type-II diabetes, as well as the inhibition of metabolism of Vitamin D (Douard et al., 2014). Vitamin D is increasingly seen as an important barrier to the reproduction of SARS-CoV-2. In order words, high levels of fructose make you more vulnerable to the virus.

If you consult your intestines, you'll find little support for sugar. Overcoming the sugar addiction requires a deeper connection with your intestines and, by developing this connection, you can develop the kind of right intuition that will better serve digestion, generally (Brown, 2016).

COVID-19 and the Stomach

There is little information about COVID-19's effect on the G.I. tract aside from its similarity to the stomach flu. To this smattering of information, I add my recent stomach-flu-like experience—that I assume was COVID-19—and my mind-body intuition.

I cannot be sure I had COVID-19 but an increasing number of healthcare practitioners, with whom I'm in contact, support the belief that many unusual illnesses over the past two months have been unrecognized cases of COVID-19. It's now acknowledged that the levels of infection were ten times what had been publicly identified, and that COVID-19 started to present itself at least a month before the illness was recognized. This information, in addition to the nature of my illness, leads me to believe I'd been "under the weather" with COVID-19 for over a month.

Two features of my G.I. experience were unusual. First, it was brief and strong. It took only four to six hours to fully manifest and caused general distress throughout my system. It manifested with diarrhea, vomiting, and a little fever the first night. This remitted the next day, during which I mostly slept, and then reappeared as serious stomach pain—like an ulcer—the second night. After 36 hours the distress diminished; I was clearly recovering after 48 hours.

The second striking effect may sound disgusting, but it was interesting at the time. The color and texture of what came out of my stomach appeared identical to what was being ejected from my colon. If you think about that, it seems impossible. I recommend using a bucket in addition to the toilet, in case that becomes relevant.

In my experience, the two substances—what comes out of the stomach and what comes from the large intestine—have little similarity. Usually, one either has trouble in the upper G.I. tract or the lower one, and they're distinct. In this case, the separation was indistinct and the experience was happening equally throughout my system. I found this reassuring, as it suggested a unified response: my system was unified in rejecting the infection.

I continued to feel weak after 48 hours as if I were not absorbing nutrients, so I purchased a middle-grade probiotic (25 billion cultures which I took twice a day) that seemed to improve my digestion and energy levels immediately.

It is now two weeks since the G.I. infection first appeared. I read that many of the COVID-19 intestinal infections metamorphose into pulmonary infections within two weeks, so I have remained concerned. I seem to be improving, though there have been a couple of days when I felt poorly.

I read that Vitamin D has a prophylactic effect (Mitchell, 2020), so I've been taking multivitamins, Vitamin D supplements, and daily walks in the sun, since the body manufactures Vitamin D using sunshine. I've continued my probiotics, a bland diet, plenty of liquids, and rest. I still feel some systemic infection hanging on in a flu-like manner. As I continue to improve two weeks after the G.I. infection, I'm confident the infection has run its course.

Stomach Teaching

I've created an induction called *The Gut Part I – Stomach* that focuses on interoception. It is not curative, and it is not designed for a person in the throes of a G.I. infection, though it might help. The induction is designed to create balance and the alliance I value and maintain between my mind and my stomach.

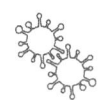

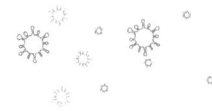

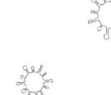

Hypnotic Session 5

The Gut Part I – Stomach audio file at:
https://www.mindstrengthbalance.com/covid19-illness-illumination/

The Gut Part I – Stomach

The Gut Part I – Stomach is a hypnotic induction that requires your full attention. Do not listen to this hypnotic visualization if you are driving a car, operating machinery, or doing anything that requires your attention.

The intention of this piece is to foster a deeper, more intuitive connection between your mind and your stomach so that you'll have greater empathy and respect for the messages, directions, and needs of your stomach.

Your stomach is only one of several organs of digestion. This piece focuses on your stomach and what it does, which is mechanically and biologically risky. While you can make intelligent decisions about what to put in your mouth, your stomach must deal with the consequences, regardless of whether or not you made the right or safe decision about what to eat.

Your stomach is a tough organ, but when it gets into trouble it needs your support, and unless you establish an intuitive connection with your stomach you will not be able to provide that support. It's the intention of this piece to educate you by opening a connection between your stomach and your mind so that you can get out of your mind, because the issues and needs of your stomach are of another world.

Begin by settling into a comfortable and relaxed position. If you're sitting, then lie back and rest your arms, neck, and head. Release the muscles that hold your frame and your posture. Start at your shoulders and relax your arms so that you can feel their weight.

Relax your chest and your ribs. Feel your ribs moving when you breathe, feel them spread with each inhale and settle with each exhale. Relax your back; this is important. Your stomach needs space, it needs to be able to move. Part of your stomach's communication with you is in its movement, so you need to feel the space it occupies.

Take a breath… inhale… and exhale. Let's count down from five so that you can give yourself a target. How you feel now is number five. And being completely relaxed is the number one. And as I count you'll feel waves of release moving through your body until I reach one and you are very relaxed, and this is just a start. You will slide more deeply into relaxation as we go on, and you will become more involved in listening and understanding the world as your stomach does.

Five, and take a deep breath, letting it out slowly.

Four, another breath, focusing on the center of your body.

Three, being aware of your lungs and the space behind them.

Two, let your mind go to the space behind your left lung.

One, inhale into this space and imagine the air going into it.

Now imagine there is a connection between your mind and your stomach. Focus on the position of your stomach within your belly. Imagine that your stomach is an organ that has abilities you don't appreciate and a purpose you don't understand. Imagine your stomach is located in your chest beneath your heart, behind your left lung. Imagine this because it's true even though you can't confirm or feel it. You have to imagine it. Your stomach is easy to imagine. You feel it all the time, you just don't notice it.

Close your eyes and relax into your stomach. Locate its position in your body, in your mind. Take a breath and fill your lungs. Notice your right lung behind your right breast, and your left lung behind the left. Move just behind your left lung and feel the space that does not expand when you inhale.

See if you can sense the shape of your stomach. Close your eyes and breath. Don't take deep breaths as they push your stomach down. Just deep enough to sense that something exists in that location, and with each breath explore this space, imagining and exploring what is a curved and flattened space. If you've eaten, the space will be larger, and if your stomach is active, the sensations will be different. If you have not eaten, this space will feel quiet.

The stomach's body is a muscle but it is unattached, so it seems separate. You cannot connect it to your spine or ribs; its mechanism and awareness are its own. It speaks a language you don't know because it is not of concepts or theories. Your stomach is the ultimate pragmatist, only concerned with what it is, and what it feels, and what it recognizes as present. And in this it establishes its moods, comfort, or satiety.

Sometimes you experience distress or some irregularity. A consciousness inclined toward action—a sense of a need to act. A more essential trust in your stomach's signals than you have in your ideas. When your stomach says, "Move," you move. Let's go toward this level of thought and feeling and see how much rapport you can build between your mind and the muscle, tissue, and nerves of your stomach.

Let's take another path to your stomach, starting in your nose and going down your throat. Inhale gently with your chest relaxed. Draw in your breath by distending your belly, drawing your lungs down. Feel the air as a weight and the more you inhale the heavier that weight gets. And this weight pulls down your eyelids and stretches out your face.

With each breath your eyelids feel heavier settling firmly shut, and your brow relaxes, pulled down by the weight. Inhale, air flowing into your belly, and pause. Feel relaxed first, and then the desire to exhale, and as you exhale you lose all sensation of your body. Inhale, and exhale.

> On the count of **one**, your head feels the passage of air going past and through your sinuses.
>
> On the count of **two**, your throat feels the passage of air like traffic under a bridge.
>
> On the count of **three**, the air diverts from your esophagus and goes down your airway.

On the count of **four**, recognize that point in your throat where your bronchi branch off and your throat continues.

On the count of **five**, imagine you leave the current of your air, but you can still hear yourself breathing.

Six, you are on your own now, moving in imagination further down your gullet.

Seven, swallow and feel the sensation of contraction riding down past where the air goes, down into that area beneath your lungs, to where your stomach is, and then the feeling disappears.

You are at the gateway to your stomach and there is a valve there. Imagine it is something like a faucet on a hose outlet. It's something that's round and fluted and it looks like it might turn, but it does not turn, and you cannot open it, at least not with force.

Imagine that you could open this valve with a password, like a magic door. All you have to do is ask it and, as if it has ears, it recognizes you. It knows who you are. You're that dull presence that rarely makes it down here, into this comfortable promised land of regular food and sustenance because you don't know anything about food, except how to eat it.

You're that lackadaisical chewer who so often sends down poorly crushed ingredients, sometimes whole tortilla chips because of your impatience and failure to really savor the taste of things. And your stomach shakes its head in dismay at your poor eating habits, and this sphincter at the top of your stomach is always the first to notice your indifference.

Let's relax further into a sense of communion with your body. You can feel yourself traveling down inside yourself, down through the tall and narrow tunnel of your throat into the darker areas. And the walls of your esophagus are moist and living. And you're surrounded by your system.

Take another breath and relax as your esophageal sphincter opens, the doorway to your stomach, and you can descend into it, like descending into a cavern from a narrow opening in the ceiling. All around you is a strange world of a thick, smooth, and ropy texture, crenelated ridges running down its length. Your stomach's lining is velvety smooth with a clear, gel coating over a shag-like carpet texture.

This is what you see, but your stomach is not a world that supports vision, it's a world that's all about preparation and recycling. Everything that comes here is taken apart, disassembled down to its molecules. This is not digestion, as that happens later, it's preparation, organization, making new packages, adding new chemicals, tearing down, neutralizing, and halting any outside, invasive process.

Your stomach is like a car wash that uses acid instead of soap. And like a car wash, it's dry until it's set into motion, at which point it floods with acids and enzymes. Filled with sensors, it feels the chemistry of everything it touches, adding just the right complements to sterilize, dissolve, and begin to break down anything digestible.

It's not at all automatic. It feels with a million fingers, and each of its muscles moves in collaboration to agitate, aggregate, palpate, mix, mash, separate, segregate, and realign. It expects what's given to it to be inert, pulverized, well-chewed, moist, soft, and passive. It has a feeding mentality, like pigs rooting through slop. Its attitude is chemical and taste is not an issue.

Your stomach loves acid, it's the only place in your body where acids are not only welcome but invited, created, distributed, and mixed into everything. It's burningly acidic there, but everywhere well-padded and protected. It feels no burn. Acid is the water of your stomach and it is most comfortable with it. And you are comfortable, insulated in a bubble of protection, in an acid car wash that would otherwise take the paint off.

Step back to sense the whole of it. Sometimes all working together with rhythms of motion. When you feel disquiet in your stomach, wrap your stomach in a gentle embrace and whisper encouragement. Settle it and see it moving in unison, gentle waves moving snail-slow across its surface. Create a cradle for it, inside your body. Rest it softly, like a cramped muscle. Massage it back to soft, back to calm, and breathe into it with reassurance.

Now imagine your stomach is having difficulty. It has noticed something there that should not be there. This could be something that just doesn't work well with the other contents, or it could be some kind of pollution, such as a bacteria. It could be that the food was bad, or it could be that some sickening agent has hitchhiked into your stomach. It could even be something you inhaled, that you've caught in the liquid lining of your mouth or nose and now have swallowed.

Your stomach is aware of these things. It does not need to wait for itself to be injured. It can sense the presence of foreign agents, and it can identify, recognize, or infer what's safe from unsafe. Some things are irritants and others may be dangerous, but either way, your stomach knows that it cannot let these things pass. It must eject them. It must send them back up and out.

Now, your stomach is acidic and this acid stays in your stomach so your mouth and throat are not familiar with this fluid. The contents of your stomach are being prepared to be torn apart and neutralized, and they are undergoing an unappetizing transformation. This material is burning, and now it needs to be sent back.

If you're insensitive to your stomach, then when your stomach needs you you'll be no more help than a child. There are things that you can do that will help your stomach, and that will help you rid yourself of what it needs to be rid of.

You can play an intelligent role in neutralizing the acid that your stomach will expel. When you feel your stomach starting to tighten you can drink a large amount of tepid, lightly salted water to dilute your stomach acid and help your stomach position exactly what it needs to remove. When you do this, you will feel your stomach relax for a moment as it receives this packaging material and begins to box up what needs to be removed. You will feel both a wider relaxation, and a smaller and more localized constriction.

Your stomach is surrounded by muscles like the arms of an octopus. It can carefully eject exactly what material it wants and it must do this quickly because this material must exit fully so you don't inhale it. The liquid is acid and it can injure your upper tissues, and it can interfere with your breathing.

The rapid heaving is what you want, and you want to support it. It does not have to be brutal or heavy-handed, it can be deft and quick, and you can help that by being relaxed and letting just those muscles that are needed perform together.

Your throat is relaxed, and your mouth, diaphragm, lungs, and tongue are relaxed. If you have swallowed warm, salted water then the material you expel will be more comfortable. And of course it will splash against your palette and behind your teeth because they are in the way. You can extend your neck and tilt your head to make the hose of your throat as straight as possible.

Remember, everything you're doing is working to get the most out, as quickly as possible, with the least effort. It is only your stomach that needs to execute the quick and forceful push, the rest of your body simply follows and responds. Your chest is relaxed, your breath is relaxed, you want to be well supported on your hands and knees or on your side. Your airways are clear, everything will flow out, and you're so relaxed that you're almost sleepy. You're so relaxed that you almost cannot feel anything.

With each contraction of your stomach you only need to exhale slightly, just enough to keep the airways clear. And after each contraction your stomach evaluates what it has done and what it further needs to do, and you know that it will be moving and reorganizing, and you are relaxed and there is no discomfort, because you are supporting the process, and the process is clearing, cleaning, and protecting you.

If necessary, you can drink more warm water because the stomach needs a flow in which to wash itself. It cannot eject if it is dry. It depends on you to serve it in this fashion, so you will have clear liquid available if your stomach needs it.

With each ejection your stomach will be feeling better, safer, and more organized. And you will know this feeling of being more settled and organized. And quite quickly you will feel relieved and relaxed until you are very relaxed, and greatly relieved, and your stomach and your whole torso are relaxed, and you have played a good role, and you have been attuned and attentive.

And after your stomach has corrected its contents it will resume its task of being on guard. A guard station that's always engaged and ready. And you will establish communications with it. Imagine there is a video connection and a phone line so that your stomach can see what you're considering, and it can speak to you over the phone to tell you what it feels. And you are sensitive, because what it tells you will be broad and complex.

Your stomach is not concerned with what tastes good, it's concerned with what is good, so its response will be settled or unsettled, cautious or welcoming, approving or hesitant. Your job is to understand these messages and to take them seriously. You will not eat just anything that presents itself. You will not eat whatever you're told to. You will consult with your stomach.

Now I'd like you to imagine that everything is normal. You have not eaten recently, your stomach may be empty or nearly so. It may have retained some food because it releases food in increments, and it retains food so that your body will have a gently varying supply. So even though you may have forgotten your last meal your stomach does not forget, and it does not hurry unless it wants to.

See in your mind's eye, or feel in your muscles, the lithe movements of your stomach, even now as it's quiet. Imagine that your stomach could purr, not a sound but a quiver, a shudder that flows over its smooth muscles, like the twitch of a horse's flank, like the flick of its tail.

Run your attention over the space where you feel your stomach lies and sense how it responds. Whenever you feel uncertainty in your gut it's either because of food or emotion.

Your stomach manages feelings and future decisions. It responds to tensions and anxieties with greater clarity than your mind, because it's not burdened with thoughts and reasons. It remembers the past as a body past. It processes hesitation and choices through a connection with memory, posture, and digestion.

Your stomach knows what's good for you, not in theory or opportunity, but right now; what really works. It weighs the toxic and the nutritive establishing a real and practical balance. This is why you must learn to hear it. Consult it like an oracle. Understand its mumblings. Its language of liquid and bubbles, twists and pulsations.

Your stomach says "good" with comfort and it can say "NO" with pains or cramps. Some of these are not problems, they are statements. If you listen to them, then they won't have to repeat themselves. If you don't listen to them, if you don't listen to your stomach, then your relationship can become distressed.

You may already have some issues of this sort, issues where you don't listen and your stomach wrestles with you. And if you listen now, and you resolve to start listening, then these issues will stop, and your relationship with your stomach—as the voice of your second brain—will move into alignment, and you will find peace, and you will find a new kind of guidance. Something intuitive, nonverbal, nonintellectual, immediate, faithful, and trusting.

Relax into your stomach. Let your breathing sit on top of your stomach. Let your stomach breathe for you.

Listen to your stomach purr as you breathe; your breath stroking down its length. And you may think this is odd, and you may think this is strange. And if you think these things, then this is a measure of how much you still are not in your stomach, but are still in your head. Hold those doubts away from you and let yourself sink into conjunction with your stomach, with the sensations of your gut.

Let your thoughts go, let them float like clouds. You've spent your whole life thinking you existed in your head and it will take time to realize there is part of you that is naturally in your gut. There is part of you that is connected to this underworld, this inner world, this world of disassembly and protection.

Scrutinizing all the parasites and pathogens that could take advantage of you, your stomach is wiser and more experienced than you are. It is the brain that is connected to your immune system, it is the seat of your immune system, it is the heart of your health and vitality. Your head is only a library and, compared to your gut, your head does little more than conducting. Your stomach is the chief engineer of the engine room and you must listen to it. But first you must hear it. You must learn to speak its language.

Now return back to the heady world of words and numbers. How far from reality of real life this is! Return to the ideas of taste and smell and touch. How far these are from nutrition and disease, good and bad bacteria, and chemistry.

Counting up and coming back out, **10**, **9**, **8**, retaining the connection, **7**, **6**, **5**, still aware of the location, **4**, **3**, **2**—back to being relaxed and reclining. Inhale… and exhale—and **one**. And when you're ready, open your eyes and be back.

7 – Time to Look Around

To regain a sense of navigating in a fluid environment.

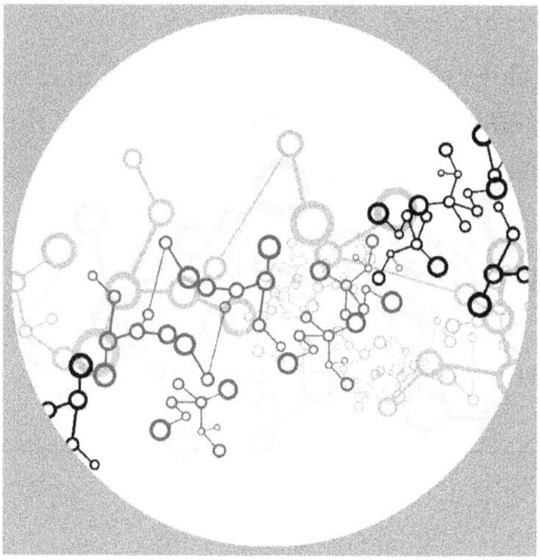

"Reject your sense of injury and the injury itself disappears."
— **Marcus Aurelius**

Questionable Information

On the world's stage are performances of failed leadership, inequitable management, poor science, and bad advice. It's not just the failure of centralized supply and distributed manufacturing, it's also the failure of centralized thinking. A failure that arises when our information and expertise is distributed by and filtered through specialists who become information bottlenecks.

The media has an average understanding of established information, but there is no established information about the virus, and the average of what's available keeps changing. Like the broken supply and manufacturing chains, the media spews questionable information like a run-away fire truck.

A critical publication on the anti-malarial drug hydroxychloroquine reported that its use in COVID-19 patients created twice as many fatalities as no treatments at all. This was widely reported by the major media and trumpeted by politicians and public health officials.

Conservative economist, Chris Martinson returned to the original research and showed, using the information in the publication, that the work was thrown together without skill or accuracy. As a result, the analysis amounted to worthless science from which no conclusions could be drawn (Martinson, 2020).

A better analysis of the data lead to a result almost contrary to what was stated and rebroadcast by the media. The study did not contradict the increasing amount of anecdotal medical literature that shows a proper administration of hydroxychloroquine had reduced serious complications from COVID-19 by almost half. In spite of this truth, the fallout effect of this fallacious report continued to mislead administrators and politicians (Risch, 2020).

When situations spin outside the norm, normal channels report information inaccurately. It is now apparent that information disseminated by two major scientific information sources, *The Lancet* and *The New England Journal of Medicine*, was compromised (Hopkins, 2020). Both journals published erroneous indications which resulted in an uproar of criticism. Both journals then retracted the two studies they'd just published.

> "My faith and trust in scientists and medical researchers and health agencies is now just broken. This is grotesque what's been happening here... I am really upset with how they have gone about everything that just happened with the Lancet trial."
>
> — **Chris Martinson**, PhD

Within days of the retraction of these studies, two different studies were published concerning the effects of hydroxychloroquine on COVID-19 patients. The first, called the RECOVERY trial, administered four times the maximum dose of this chemical to extremely ill patients. Both the trial and the control groups experienced statistically indistinguishable 24% mortality, give or take one percent. The trial was not completed but, nevertheless, the authors concluded the drug had no beneficial effect under any circumstances.

The second study (Boulware et al., 2020) gave hydroxychloroquine to subjects who were thought to have been exposed to the virus and found that it did not alter the percentage of those who were eventually diagnosed with the illness. They were not able to determine which subjects were or were not infected with the virus, and none of the statistics accounted for the large effect this had on their results. The consequence of this was that their actual sample size was small. They also concluded, with slightly more reservation, that the chemical offered no benefit.

Neither study addressed the phase of early infection during which clinicians were finding the chemical to be effective. From our understanding of the role of hydroxychloroquine in the metabolism of the cell, the chemical's effect is to impede the reproduction of the virus. It has no effect on the virus's ability to infect a person, or the recuperative power of a severely sick patient.

While the results are interesting, we would not have expected this chemical to be effective in either situation. The studies were irrelevant. In addition, the excessive dose used in the RECOVERY trial appears to have been assigned through the mistake of confusing hydroxychloroquine with Hydroxyquinoline, an unrelated substance (Citizen's Collective, 2020).

Both studies addressed the wrong question. Both studies made sweeping, unjustified conclusions that are now being accepted by healthcare administrators and grant funding organizations. As a result, funding, interest, and research in understanding hydroxychloroquine's potentially beneficial effect are coming to a halt.

Doctor Scientists

Doctors make terrible scientists. This is widely recognized and further demonstrated by these comic, tragic, and misguided studies.

Doctors are not trained in science. They have no time to be scientists and gain little benefit from collecting, collating, and correcting large quantities of data. They are trained to be inductive and not deductive. They risk professional censure and disciplinary action if they deviate from standard practice. They are required to think inside the box of accepted practice, and they are legally liable for making the kinds of mistakes that science depends on.

Doctors are personally, professionally, and institutionally subsidized by the pharmaceutical industry which subjects them to heavy advertizing. They are unschooled in statistics, unpracticed in disciplines outside their field, and increasingly unskilled in the collection and study of individual patient histories.

Under normal circumstances, these deep and indicting failures are somewhat offset by careful editing, fact-checking, and scientific scrutiny. None of that is happening at this time. The result is that erroneous, compromised, and manipulated medicine is being accepted as science which is forming the basis for public policy and future research.

You must gather information yourself. The information you need is available. To become informed, first recognize that being informed is not your right, it's your responsibility.

> "Governments and official bodies didn't seem to be very proactive about (educating people about COVID-19) so I made videos to get people to get thinking about it. I'm surprised it has become so popular, but clearly there is a thirst for information."
>
> — **Dr. John Campbell**

Do not rely on the major media, politicians, or public health officials who are answerable to vested interests. For these people the balance of power is primary and truth is secondary. Instead, follow individual doctors and scientists who are accurate observers. Here are three sources of accurate medical and statistical information who post regular, free, instructional videos.

John Campbell, PhD:
https://www.youtube.com/channel/UCF9IOB2TExg3QIBupFtBDxg

Chris Martenson, PhD:
https://www.peakprosperity.com/

Roger Seheult, MD:
https://www.medcram.com/

The mainstream media is a narcotic cocktail of irrelevant spectator sports, palliative social bonding, and damaging misinformation. Listening to mainstream media is like huddling on the Titanic and listening to clueless leadership while select elements of the corporate infrastructure lower financial bailout lifeboats to first-class passengers. We must take responsibility for being informed using both original sources and our bodies' wisdom.

Future Management

Successful planning is not built solely on an intellectual understanding of the situation. If we take that approach, then our course is optimized by learning all the facts, and it only changes when the facts change. This strategy works when the facts are known, the goal is fixed, the path evident, and our intentions are clear. In business, this static approach is called "the waterfall approach" because once we begin, we're inexorably swept over the consequences like a series of waterfalls.

The requirements of this approach are rarely met. In a changing world, it does not make sense to fix a method for a creative process. Every ingredient of the waterfall approach is subject to change and the larger, longer, or more complex the project, the greater the number of its elements that may change with time or context. We're in the middle of a complex project now: the pandemic.

In organizations, the waterfall approach fails more than 75% of the time. It fails because organizations are dissociated personalities that rely on numbers. They lack a connection with their subconscious and have no intuition to guide them. They are the organizational equivalent of insane people.

People don't organize their lives using the waterfall approach, though they give it lip service. It sounds good to say we've got it figured out, but, in fact, the more well-balanced we are, the less structure we need.

Well-balanced people intuit the stability and solidity of their environment. At the same time, the more our environment loses its stability and solidity, the less well-balanced we become. Figuring our way forward through uncertain times requires greater personal flexibility, stability, and insight than normal.

The insight we need is both insight into external events and insight into the needs and motivations of people, including ourselves. Our own needs become difficult to manage when the needs in our environment lose form: we are the stories we tell.

These are times to find and hold our center, both individually and collectively. Community cohesion is both a social and a personal need. Politicians and administrators who fail to create unity are either personally dysregulated or are looking for personal profit.

Simply arguing for personal balance does not make it happen. It may turn your attention inward, but it's not clear that you'll know what to do with what you see. This is a circumstance where what we call management morphs into what we call therapy. Management is always more than just arranging the pieces, and therapy is more than fixing what's broken.

Project Therapy

I suggest a session with your subconscious. Your subconscious is your silent partner, except it's not so silent when your personality cracks. Then, the sea of emotional perception and emotional expression inundates your landscape.

There are three situations in which you're in deeper touch with your subconscious: in your feelings, in your dreams, and at some fundamental level all the rest of the time.

In the last of these—during "all the rest of the time"—your subconscious streams behind you. You're looking forward into the "real world" like a person running a race, focusing on the image of progress. Considering your subconscious in these situations takes finesse lest it causes you to stumble. This is why the subconscious is ignored in business: it's too amorphous and complex.

Your dreams have been reminding you of your subconscious's presence in your daily life. Dreams inject fertile chaos: the uncertainty of unconsidered possibilities. Dreams are disruptive elements from your subconscious, more disruptive than what's already on your radar.

Dreams emerge to have disruptive effects if you have the mental resources they require. You'll have dreams even if you lack these resources, but you won't remember them. In that case, their operation will remain in your subconscious, lost from recollection.

Your feelings are invitations to consciously engage the currents of your subconscious. The feelings of others are opportunities for building consensus. Feelings are the dumplings in the stew of your emotions. Moods are the perceptual gloss these emotions caste on the world around you. Urges are the ideas that bubble up.

To invite your subconscious, sink into your feelings. Explore your moods and let your urges speak to you. Engage your emotions like a wobbly landlubber boarding a sailboat, fumbling to cast-off, and let the wind carry you.

I've written the guided visualization called *The Voyage* to trace the steps from the conscious to the subconscious. *The Voyage* builds a cross-dimensional bridge between the apparently definitive conscious world and the soft, multi-layered subconscious world from which we create our conscious perception.

The goal is to navigate in the current, chaotic environment: lowering the keel of emotional balance and raising the sail of intuition to move with direction through your fluid situation. The visualization uses a land-ocean-boat metaphor. It doesn't require that you have boating experience. In fact, it's better if you don't. That way, what you imagine will be your mind's real territory, not one from memory. Join me in *The Voyage*.

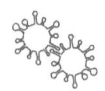

Hypnotic Session 6

The Voyage audio file at: https://www.mindstrengthbalance.com/covid19-illness-illumination/

The Voyage

The Voyage is a hypnotic induction that requires your full attention. Do not listen to this hypnotic visualization if you are driving a car, operating machinery, or doing anything that requires your attention.

Begin by imagining you've lived all your life on land. All your life you've explored a solid landscape with nothing more yielding than an lounge chair or mud puddle. With the exception of a few slippery steps, your life has moved forward along paths of wood, stone, earth, carpet, or concrete, rough or smooth. You are a person who stands by feeling your feet, creating your legs and then, like building a snowman, you place your body on top. Grounding to you, for all your life, has meant contact with the ground.

Relax now. Settle down and let gravity take you as close to the ground as you can go, resting every part of youself on a settled surface. Your feet, your thighs, butt, and back, shoulders, arms, hands, and head. Throughout all of our lives our feet are on something, feeling down to something incompressible, the solidity of our identity.

Take a breath and notice how your inhale lifts you up. It lifts you away from your feet, almost into your imagination. Like a periscope, your inhale lets shafts of light in from somewhere, a break in the clouds, a foreign breeze, a momentary imbalance. It's necessary in order to get a better grip.

And when you exhale you settle and things shift and you become wrapped up in yourself. Like a landslide settling, your exhale brings all the movements together and then, at the very bottom, everything settles.

With your next inhale you feel like a balloon rising from a slab of slate;

you feel both the slate and the balloon rising on their own powers into an airy world of novelty and aspiration. Now exhale… now inhale. At the top of your inhale you want to feel fulfilled. Nothing else; no thoughts, no words nor sentences, just completion.

Notice that when you do speak or think, it's this sense of completion that's always your goal. Regardless of what you're speaking or thinking about, it's the feeling of finishing the thought that attracts you like a summit. And if it takes several thoughts or sentences to get there, then the thought is "complete," and for a moment we feel complete, and that's a feeling you love, balanced for a moment with nothing more to say.

Sometimes we arrive at thoughts that are so well finished and complete that there is no more. So often this escapes us, but imagine life was so simple and straightforward that after every exhale there was nothing more to say or think. All that's left to pass through your mind are scraps and left-over words that evaporate like clouds. Inhale with a sense of having something to say… and exhale with the feeling of it all being said: all said and done. Inhale into that feeling of openness… and exhale into completion.

Now the world is disrupted, and this extends beyond your own smaller world. What do you know of its disruption? Have you really experienced it? Could you, or is it just an idea? Some people have suffered, others are in suspense, left to imagine what might be, what might have been, and what is to come.

Relax your body. Focus on those joints and muscles where you store your tension, like the larder where you keep your canned goods. I invite you on a journey on foot, and you can leave the canned goods behind. Take a last look in those closets, just to make sure everything is there, and close the cupboards. Go through each of your stores of tension, arrange them as needed, and let them go. You won't need them.

Inhale into the cabinets of your incompletions, and close them with your exhale. Put their tensions aside, let them go: your neck, your left shoulder, and then your right shoulder, your upper back, your lower back, diaphragm, hips.

Release the tension in your left knee and then your right knee. Your left ankle and then your right ankle. Your left foot and then your right foot. Your left wrist and left hand, and then your right wrist and right hand.

Feel the weight of your left arm and your left elbow and let these sink down into whatever supports them. Move to your right arm and your right elbow. Let these sink down into whatever supports them. Becoming more relaxed in your body and your mind with each breath.

Leave your body as a container and rise to stand above it. Imagine your arms hanging by your sides and your feet beneath your shoulders. Imagine raising your elbows, lifting your hands in front of your face with your arms bent. Unfold your arms, straightening them to point away, raising your arms above your head.

Imagine there is no stress, or strain, or weight: as light as a feather. Slowly lower your arms and feel yourself in the best of health, balanced, sensitive, aware, and strong. You have no soreness or resistance. Your motion is smooth and effortless. Try walking and feel it move through you like a wave. You can even run and it feels like floating, there is no impact, only a rolling, balanced motion.

Take this virtual sense of self and place, and move into your imagined landscape. You are emerging from a warm and well-stocked cottage in the country. Wide French doors open into an organized and exuberant garden of shining green leaves, white flowers, and moss-covered stones, ringed by small trees and a low, vine-covered fence. And you walk through this garden, almost able to hear the conversations between the plants.

You reach the gate and stop and look back. The garden is compact and joyful, everything in its place and growing within its bounds. Alive, vibrating in colors, small movements and sounds. Behind you is the gate to the outside where there is trouble. Some people are sick and some are dying in a new environment whose change has been microscopic. And we used to scoff at the plagues of the middle ages because they didn't know what germs were and we do, but we're hardly any better for knowing it.

And you know these things will disturb the order and progress of the garden as it does take tending, care, resources, and attention, and now you are distracted and everyone is distracted, and resources won't be as available as before, and you'll have to do other things.

Take a breath and go deeper, 3, 2, 1, down into the porous rock. Down into the slow flow of the groundwater that migrates down into the aquifer and out into the sea. The plasma of the land bearing the nutrients along with roots and roads and rain.

You are out in the world now, in the community, on the familiar streets with a certain denial. The changes are temporary, you tell yourself. The shuttered shops seem like they just closed and will soon reopen. Some windows are papered over and you put those out of your mind as if they're just part of the background.

Some things were weak before and now, most likely they'll be gone. Expensive specialty stores selling things for people who had the money for everything and still more. There are new services. The homeless are now gathered, tended to, and less in need. And you tell yourself these are temporary, soon to return to how it was before, to maybe new and better ways.

There is a nervousness and uncertainty; a wonderland of talk and planning. Lots of collaboration and support from people who have not been collaborative or supportive. New friends by necessity and old ones unavailable.

Close your eyes and sink into the earth, like a tree's energy sinks into its roots, the energy of a field of tulips, or a root-entangled forest. Your roots are everywhere, and you can move from place to place by just being there because you understand the energy is everywhere, and all places are connected. Feel connected to these places.

The news is the same everywhere, the concerns are the same everywhere, people are feeling the same everywhere. You are in none of these places and you are in all of them.

You listen to a rhythm of uncertainty and dislocation that resonates like a sounding board through the collected minds, across countries, continents, and cultures. And you hear voices of strife and recrimination rattle like buzzing strings, downed power lines short-circuiting, that attack the culture, drain power, feed on fear in a search for opportunity.

It's an earthquake of group thinking, it's hard to stand upright, it knocks you down. There is nothing in its place to nourish or direct. Social isolation is like a cultural fast. The culture ridding itself of sickness by halting its function, freezing in place, to halt the peristalsis of money, trade, construction, transportation, travel, art, expression, and all our habits needed, unneeded, and unaware.

Just relax and let these thoughts parade on past like a bad marching band, shrill, cacophonous, and dissonant. Settle back to your roots. Inhale… exhale… Down to quiet in your thoughts. Down to ground level like a puddle on the earth. Down deeper into the earth with fingers through the soil. Down into the water table moving toward the ocean.

Time passes. People talk. Some get sick, some get better. Some go into crisis and prevail or succumb. The blue sky is filled with a patchwork of holes and the groundwater moves to the sea. Some of it finds streams and rivers, most of it percolates slowly over weeks and months.

And now you are at the sea, and that is a different world, and you draw back from its formlessness, from the booming sounds inside it. The water has no points, no landmarks, no fixed point of reference. Beyond the shore, beyond the seabed, the water speaks only to itself.

You are at the seashore by a sailboat. Maybe it's a small boat or maybe it's a big one. Maybe you have to push it into the surf, or maybe you're on a dock and you can step onto it. And it's floating and tied to the shore, maybe to a cleat on the dock, or a tree on the beach. And the boat notices you and reacts as you move. And the water notices you, too, and you and the boat and the water are all one affair.

You're part of a shifting form whose balance is searching for a center. Unlike the shore where all forces fix upon the ground, here the forces are always juggling, looking for a way to put down the heavy things, as if the water is always tired of carrying it.

You wiggle and the boat wiggles, and the water wiggles, and you hear the water say, "You are a visitor. All visitors are welcome. There is always space. There is always rhythm. Everything is in communication. Join the conversation." So you do, and you sit down, and you cast off the line, pulling it into the boat, pulling the last straight thing that holds you to the land and now you can start to speak the rhythms of the sea.

Raise your sail into the ocean of the air with its currents and waves, transparent sounds and lack of surfaces. And you are to travel between these states of matter, wedged between the water and the air, each twisting you in different ways, like two hands working to unscrew a jar, but you hold together, and the hand of water and the hand of air slip over your surface and you pop forward, like a lemon seed.

Here is space, but also no space. Without the shore, everywhere is the same with only your process changing, the process of movement and sensation. Out of sight of land you feel the water rumble and the air hum and all the chaos of the waves of the oceanic and aerial worlds. You are nowhere and everywhere, feeling waves that have bounced from distant shores mixed with the tumult of windswept spray.

Like the disturbed culture, the wind talks incessantly of the weather, yet never does anything about it. It's not even cause and effect, it's just effect, just like the culture bemoaning its lack of control, unable to ride over nature as has been our habit. Like people on a stranded boat pulling, pulling, pulling at the starter cord of their outboard motor, paying no attention to the language of the sea and the sky. But you are not on that boat, your boat has a sail above and a keel below, a sail slipping between the fingers of the elements.

Relax and let your mind drift. Separate your mind from the frustrating talk of control and prediction. All of the future and the past are in the air and ocean currents. You are not fasting in isolation, you are listening to the lapping of the future on the hull of your boat. And the boat is your body and your mind and your feeling. And the boat is your culture and your country and your business. It is your family and your neighborhood which lap against you like the small waves, and the larger swells are the waves of talk and action, agitated molecules that hum and whip and snap the sails.

Don't listen to this language, listen to the waves. Listen into the waves for meanings and connections; the changing rhythms, not the clicks and snaps. Feel for the texture, not the threads. The song of the virus is not in the notes, it's in the melody, something bigger than the ears of others, but you can hear it.

Take a breath, and as your inhale ends let it keep going in your mind, like the waves that keep radiating outward from the stone. Your exhale is just the quiet inside the circle and it too, radiates outward. Inhale with the drop of another stone… and exhale into the quiet circle of water within its growing radius.

That is your breath, a series of circles that keep on going, traveling across the ocean, and they'll get dimmer and larger with time and distance but they'll never stop. If you were on land they would leave no trace beyond your body, but here in the ocean, they join the concern of all the actions on the surface.

Listen for the breathing of the others, the discord and the fears. With your mind, answer them with consonance. Guide them all to resonance. It's easy: simply receive their energy and hold it until your next exhale. Then let it go. Listen with your eyes, hold them with your ears, and guide them with your breath.

You can be here anytime you like. You can help others find the rhythmic waves not by telling or talking, but by being part of them. By joining your breath with your attention, fixed on the energy of others, you bring them into alignment with the waves around us.

Moving through an ocean of possibility, leaving behind the foamy wake of consternation. Leaving all the chaos of strife and struggle to settle back into the ocean behind us. Trust the forces that move us forward. Synchronize with them, like a meditation, like a choir, like the breathing of the culture. Inhale… exhale… Inhale… exhale...

8 – Future Visions

Exploring the idea that our mind has the power to affect our membranes.

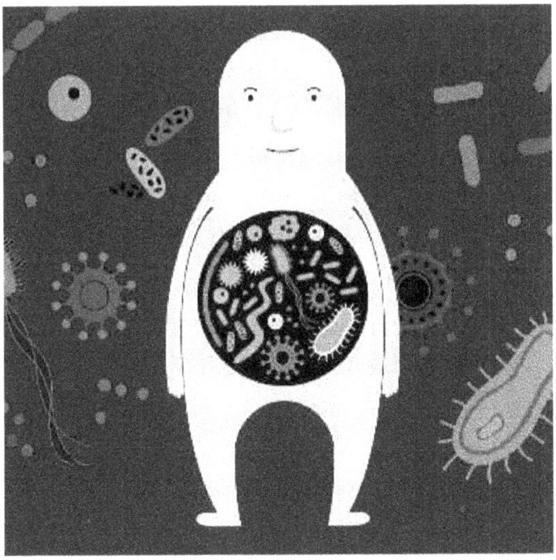

"The 'Heart of Energy Medicine' may truly be found in the magic of the membrane."
—**Bruce Lipton**, PhD

Partners

The battle for your health is not about herd immunity or vaccination, it's about which of your cells live and which die. It's a fight for who wins in the present, but it's also for the future. It's a struggle between species.

If this battle seems new, that's because our lives are short. The virus is the reproductive organ of an older, quasi-life form whose history spans the lineage of its identity. It has no body, organs, digestive system, or central nervous system, but it does have a plan. It reproduces by finding energy and opportunity without bothering to stop and evolve into life as we know it.

Rather than support a body, a metabolism, organs to create a flower and seed, the virus has reduced itself to just a seed which finds ways to reproduce in other organisms. It is a seed with instructions, and nothing more: the simplest, most primitive, efficient, self-reproducing form of all. In spite of this, the virus has evolved a technology beyond anything we can match.

You live in a body, an identity, a legacy, a family, culture, country, and economy. You have built patterns, memories, discoveries, and creations. The virus has none of those but somehow, by investing everything in its environment, it has found hosts for all of those, piggy-backing on whatever its host species has developed. And the more productive, robust, creative, successful, and adventurous the host, the greater the benefit the virus finds for itself.

Wherever you go, whatever you do, however much you accomplish, the virus will tag along with its singular focus: to multiply. And if you learn how to remove, deny, or overcome it, it simply diminishes in you and prevails elsewhere. Moving, settling, multiplying, and moving again. It can grow without bounds or hide in the smallest retreat to wait for a new carrier, home, or opportunity.

Perils

At the turn of the 19th century, science stimulated our imagination to explore new realms: beneath the earth, under the sea, and beyond the sky. Hidden lairs for hidden threats: cavemen, sea monsters, and little green men. We imagined them big because bigger is scarier, but the ancient lairs are small—at the roots, not the peaks of evolution.

These evolutionarily distant life forms are both threats and partners, in the same way that without fungus nothing would decay, without insects the food chain would collapse, without plankton we'd suffocate, without bacteria we'd starve.

And what of viruses—what role do they play? Every time we've dismissed or abused some element of our ecology we've suffered harsh consequences. Anything that's pervasive plays a major role, whether we understand the formula or not.

Viruses are arguably our oldest partners. Are they parasites or saprophytes?

They assail our immunity, but they have brought us DNA. At its most basic level, life is survival and reproduction, and all that we know about survival—our immunity to anything—has been taught to us by viruses. If you can't beat 'em, join 'em.

> "Whatever their origin, viruses have played a central role in evolution. They may have enabled the transition from a primordial RNA world to the modern DNA world. The nucleus of eukaryotic cells may have started life as a parasitic virus. And virus genes that integrated into their hosts' genomes introduced many evolutionary novelties; for example, the ERVW-1 gene that plays a central role in the formation of the mammalian placenta is viral in origin. We may fear and loathe viruses—especially right now—but without them we would not be here."
>
> — **Graham Lawton** (2020), in "Viruses: Viruses are the most abundant organisms on Earth, and probably played a pivotal role in the origin of life", in *New Scientist.*

> "Viruses seem to be ubiquitous and have been reported from any environment where life is present, from fresh waters to the sands of the Sahara desert. However, very little is known of the ecological roles of viruses in most ecosystems… There may be at least 1000 different viruses living in the human gut. The vast majority, over 70%, of genetic material carried by these viruses is completely uncharacterized, and natural viral communities probably represent the largest unexplored area of genetic information space left on the planet."
>
> — **Rohwer, Prangishvili, & Lindell** (2009), in "Roles of viruses in the environment."

Membranes

Our cell membranes make us separate, acting as organizers, enforcers, and arrangers; they may even be the brains behind much of life. Beyond all the bluster and battleground, the buck stops at the cell's membrane.

Beneath the talk of contagion and cure, it's the virus's ability to open the membrane that makes all the difference. This process of opening a door is neither a contest nor a battle; it's a quiet, careful process that either works perfectly or not at all.

Like the membrane of our skin, our cell walls pass many messages but admit no visitors. These walls have many doors, all of which are locked, but there are keys. If you break into the cell without the key, alarms go off and the immune system attacks you.

Among our membrane's many locks is one called ACE2, an acronym for the angiotensin molecule that spans the membrane's width. The key to ACE2 is a protein that fits with it—the key to the lock—that opens a molecule-sized doorway.

This is a complicated key, with thousands of precisely located atoms in a specific protein. There is not just one ACE2 key, but many possible ones, with some working better than others.

The virus has an ACE2 key; its surface is studded with duplicates. They are the protein spikes that give the virus a crown-like appearance. The key carried by the SARS-CoV-2 virus is particularly good at unlocking the cell membrane, binding ten to twenty times more tightly to the ACE2 lock than the keys of previous corona viruses (Wrapp et al., 2020).

Protein Keys

Carried randomly through our system, floating on whatever currents we create in ourselves, the virus is a beggar tick catching on any of the billion ACE2 locks that adorn the walls of our cells. Its key opens a small door, a molecule-sized mail slot, and through this mail slot the virus sends a blank message whose contents, much like an email virus we might receive, says nothing. As a result, the cell doesn't realize it's been compromised and does not react. But this message has an attachment, and once inside the cell, this attachment opens.

The attachment contains the virus's RNA along with certain chemical instructions. In a process below the level of life, these instructions attract natural chemicals within the cell's cytoplasm and place them in positions necessary to begin the process of copying the virus's RNA.

We don't know how this process works to create an exact copy of the whole, semi-living virus, just as we don't know how our cells form and reform themselves. This is not a process controlled by DNA; it's much more complicated. We have no clear idea of what controls it.

Within a few hours, thousands of viral copies have been made and our cell bursts, spewing thousands of new virions, or virus particles, into our intercellular liquids. When that happens, our body knows it's under attack and begins a general process of chemical, cellular, metabolic defense, some of which target invaders, shut down normal metabolism, and even attack itself. A massive conflagration begins.

Very much like a war between humans, whatever risk the invaders impose can be made much worse by the widespread decimation that occurs in response to that risk. Some of us, it seems, choose the "nuclear option" and, as a result, kill ourselves in the process.

At first, we thought COVID-19 was a lung disease, but it turns out the virus can reproduce in practically any cell that it can get into, which is any cell that has the ACE2 lock embedded in its membrane.

If we inhale COVID-19, it attaches to cells in our respiratory tract. If we ingest it, it will attach in our digestive tract; and if it gets into our bloodstream, it may attach to cells in any of a range of organs, including our skin, bone marrow, spleen, liver, kidney, and brain, as well as the cells lining all of our veins and arteries (Hamming et al., 2004).

The virus likely reaches our lungs first, but young people, who don't tend to show symptoms in their lungs, are showing symptoms in their skin. And some are experiencing an infection in other organs weeks after recovering from an infection in their lungs. Our bodies do not have a unified response.

Protecting the Boundary

It seems inconceivable that through the power of the mind alone we can micromanage our white blood cells, but we can. Through force of mind alone we can raise or lower our white blood cell count. More than that: we can change their relative numbers within our blood to raise or lower the ratio of neutrophils to leukocytes.

We don't know how this is done; we don't even know which ratio is best, yet somehow we can do it. What of the other minority types of white blood cells, the basophils, eosinophils, monocytes, B cells, T cells, and killer cells? Can we change the ratios of their population in our blood, too?

Let's go a step further to the molecular level. Can our minds control the biochemistry of our membranes? We don't know how this is done at any level, even within the cell's chemistry, yet here is the root of our vulnerability and the key to our protection.

I have created a hypnotic visualization called *Membrane Locksmith* that explores the idea that our mind has the power to affect our membranes. I don't know of any direct evidence to suggest we can do this, but, until recently, I didn't know of the evidence that through force of mind we could alter our white blood cell counts. It's an experiment.

> "The nervous system translates consciousness into blood chemistry, which in turn, directly shapes the epigenetic fate of our cells. These cellular mechanisms represent the molecular master switches through which thoughts, attitudes, and beliefs create the conditions of our body."
>
> — **Bruce Lipton**, PhD, from "Crisis Ignites Evolution"

> "The commonly held perception is that your genes are a blueprint of your life —this is totally false. The blueprint of your life is based on your perception, because your genes will change according to your perceptions."
>
> — **Bruce Lipton**, PhD, from "The Jump From Cell Culture to Consciousness" (Gustafson, 2017)

Hypnotic Session 7

Membrane Locksmith file at: https://www.mindstrengthbalance.com/covid19-illness-illumination/

Membrane Locksmith

Membrane Locksmith is a hypnotic induction that requires your full attention. Do not listen to this hypnotic visualization if you are driving a car, operating machinery, or doing anything that requires your attention.

In 2012 the geneticist Bruce Lipton said, "When I have a thought, my mind sends out signals, in the form of growth factors, hormones, or other chemicals. Thoughts can also initiate rapid oscillations of nerve cells... signals sent out by your central nervous system actually override the function of cell membrane receptors... responding to signals in their immediate environment... the brain can ultimately control the activity of tissues and organs... (and) actually influence the membrane."

Bruce Lipton suggests our thoughts control our metabolism to levels we have not explored. There are stories of unexplained healings, and careful attention has provided new reports, some well substantiated but still unexplained. We don't know how it's done and we don't know the mind's limits. It seems to be a skill that builds with practice, which only makes it more difficult to understand.

In this visualization, you'll explore the idea of creating intentions to guide your cells. The world of cells is foreign and complex, a chemical world we don't experience directly, but a viral infection may offer an exception. A perfect crisis and opportunity.

Viruses have figured out how to unlock our cells, getting through the cell's membrane by stealth and deception. We know the science behind their strategy, but our cells can't recognize the deceit. We would like to tell our cells what's happening, but they speak a chemical language. Can we say or think or feel something that our cells will hear?

We'll relax our minds to become as attentive as possible to feelings, sensations, and insight. Everything we do here, and anything we can accomplish, requires a deeper level of connection. Deeper than your thinking mind, your talking self, even your sense of self. If you know how to be present in a trance, go there. If you don't, then become absent, find the feeling of going to sleep.

Find a comfortable position where you can lean back and let your body relax. Settle into your bed, sofa, chair, or recliner and consciously relax your arms and shoulders. Take a deep breath and follow how your feeling changes as your lungs inflate. As you exhale, feel your neck and torso relax and your mind release, becoming less attached and less fixed.

Your body is like a small pond. You are at the center and feel the edges all around you. The edges are your skin and what touches them sends ripples across the surface. The pond's edge wraps around as your sense of your own boundary wraps around you. Just as a pebble dropped in the center radiates waves to the shoreline, so your pulse moves through your body, not feeling everywhere all at once, but wherever you focus and settle into it. Your heart's beat is a pulse of awareness that activates all your cells like a distant drumbeat.

Settle into your pulse. Imagine your heart beats to the rhythm of the little ripples at the edge of the pond, ripples so small you cannot even hear them. Imagine all the sound in your pulse, and you can feel it if you quiet your senses. You can sense it in any part of your body that you focus on, and you can feel if it's calm and smooth, or uneven and irregular, and whatever you feel, you can make that feeling calmer and smoother.

Settle down to the microscopic level where everything is liquid. Our bodies are an ocean of moving nutrients, like black smokers on the sea bed pouring nutrients from unseen sources, coming into us from the outside world to circulate through our arteries. And what lives inside us, all of our cells and organs, they don't know, they take it for granted like shoals of fish and sea anemones. They move as they will and survive on what comes past.

But then, we take what we have for granted, too.

Count your way down to a lower level of awareness. Use your breath and its connection to your heart. Sense your pulse within your breath. Feel it at the top of your breath as it floats up like a dark and hidden fish, to sink down again with your exhale. Let it rise with your inhale and fall as you count down from five.

> Counting **five**, inhale and look into the pond, and exhale as the shadow of your pulse recedes again.
>
> **Four**, inhale into the pulse, as the elusive pulse returns, and exhale tipping forward into your relaxation.
>
> **Three**, inhale and see the shape of your pulse, and exhale feeling that shape repeat.
>
> **Two**, and now you can sense other things, like shapes in shadows fading as you exhale.
>
> **One**, the image of a rising fish, a heightened sense, a fading awareness with your slow exhale.

Emotions affect our cells, and in ways we can steer our cells precisely, but we don't know how we do it. Consider imagination as a language whose metaphors translate into the language of our cells.

Simplify your feelings, to project these feelings onto another context. Relax into a place of imagination. Imagine you can feel memories and images as they really were. Your mirror of the past is just as clear and is the present again. Just as you can think of a lemon to make your mouth water, you can think of things that trigger sensations in your body.

Inhale feeling satisfied, as nothing else is needed as your thoughts get smaller. Release these thoughts with your exhale and let background ideas fall away. Clear your palette of tastes, your air of sounds, and your canvas of images.

Your eyes are closed, your body is warm, your thoughts are heavy, getting heavier, slower, lower, settling too heavy, too heavy to lift, so you lift off from them to move through new, light thoughts with barely any substance.

You're in a warm shower and your inhale wrings out a big sponge. On your exhale you're wiping tensions off your arms, shoulders, and sides. Washing them away. Your inhale is the hot water massaging your skin with heat and sensation, and your exhale is the water flowing to spread warmth, washing across your skin creating a current.

Imagine you have shrunk to the size of a cell in your body, and your body is the size of a cell, and you're aware of the skin of your cell like the skin of your body. There are so many sensations across your skin that you barely notice them. Sometimes there is an itch or a scratch, a spot, a flash, or a poke. You might flinch but not think much of it. You might move but you hardly think about it.

Imagine the virus is the size of a potato chip, and you eat potato chips all the time, and you never think about it, you just eat them whenever you encounter them. It's a habit, a routine, a compulsion.

But these potato chips are not the same. They look the same and taste the same, but there's something wrong with them. You have to know in your mind that you don't want them because in other regards they seem like all the rest. They would trigger you and you would eat them, but now the idea has come to you that you should not, that you don't want to, and with a change of attitude you impose your willpower to stop yourself. You don't let them in. You don't follow your habit. You're feeling differently.

Suppose you are the cell and you do a kind of breathing, of taking in and letting out. And cells do that, taking in oxygen and sugars and releasing carbon dioxide and water. Imagine that there is a dust in the oxygen you breathe, it's like a pollen and you notice it but you might not do anything about it.

This pollen, this dust, is different. Its particles are the virus. It's toxic and you must not take it in. You are aware that this dust carries a sickness and you don't want to breathe it in. Imagine you could put up a barrier, maybe your cells can breathe more carefully, or breathe as if wearing a mask, or filter with greater care, to be vigilant.

This might interfere with how you function. It might slow your response and disrupt things. You might become hungry or your thinking clouded. To become careful and defensive you need a higher level of awareness and control.

Accept and feel this responsibility as a felt sense, a warmth or energy. Move this sense of warmth and care into your tissues, a sense of care that you can feel in your muscles as a relaxed energy. Move this sensation into your skin, the bones of your torso and spine, into the bone marrow and into your heart.

You'll have to communicate with other processes, other cells and chemical processes. Many things may need to reorganize, like people keeping their distance, shepherding their resources, limiting their consumption, and rearranging their lives.

You might feel tired, dull, or achy. You might feel moody or agitated. Take all these as possibilities and welcome them as a healing state, not as problems. Feel these as consequences of drawing in, stepping back, being cautious and selective. Let yourself slow down and spend this extra energy to protect yourself.

You can watch these things, these new characters and actions, and just let them play out. Your slow or cranky self may even be better than your normal self at discriminating and dealing with the delays and challenges. If you feel less compassionate and welcoming, you may be more disciplined and circumspect. Your boundary is thicker and harder, and your inclination is to slow down commerce, intercourse, and dialog of all kinds.

You cannot see your cells directly, you don't know what they see and the decisions they make. They hold no conversation you can hear. But they do communicate and you don't know because you can't find them as parts of yourself.

Imagine you are aware of the communications between your cells. It is a sound in the background that comes with a feeling and a sense. Listen to it now, not just to the nerves going to and fro between different cells, but to the chemistry of minerals and nutrients, water, gasses, light and darkness. Listen to the feelings in your body.

Relax more deeply. Move from a consciousness of one to a consciousness of many, to collective feeling and collective thought. Take a breath and sink into a state of sleep, directing all of your attention to within yourself. The voices in your head are too shrill, too declarative, too opinionated.

You haven't found it. Your thinking is too thin, make it thicker, deeper. Inhale and count backwards by hundreds, starting at five hundred and going back one hundred at a time:

> Inhale… Exhale: **five hundred**, sinking deeper, getting softer, more relaxed.
>
> Inhale… Exhale: **four hundred**, deeply relaxed, feeling currents deep in your muscles.
>
> Inhale… Exhale: **three hundred**, and your hands and feet are heavy, wrapped in energy.
>
> Inhale… Exhale: **two hundred**, thinking of cells, a spreading, collective awareness.
>
> Inhale… Exhale: **one hundred**, your pulse is steady, breathing easier, and sensations calm.
>
> Inhale… Exhale: **zero**, all awareness inside you, a new city, a new domain, all sensitivity, no speech, all listening, no thinking, all sensing through signals and associations.

You are a world of cells, four thousand times as many as there are people in the world. Consider a small collection of cells, perhaps a thousand or ten thousand, all inhabitants of your body, all part of a neighborhood. They don't need discussions; they hear thoughts and work together.

Your single thought can speak for them all, for the whole tissue. Your single thought can speak to them, all hearing you as one mind. Your one sensation can be shared by every cell. Maybe it's a sense of caution, rest, or restraint. The cells speak to you as one voice, as one sensation, insight, or inspiration shared by all cells as a group-mind: care, defense, protection, strength, healing, and support.

You are your skin, your whole envelope, a container covering all of you, all one organ. Your mind speaks to all your skin as through a loudspeaker creating a thin wave reverberating across your surface. The message is to bolt the doors, check every visitor's credentials. Don't leave the neighborhood unattended. Ill weeds grow fast.

Now you are your circulatory systems, extending out as miles of arteries and veins. Big arteries like pipelines and little passageways, hardly one cell wide which guide currents of nutrients and chemicals, and may float a million viruses.

If we inhale them, they enter our respiratory tract. If we ingest them, they enter our digestive tract. And if they get into our bloodstream, though not with our permission, they can travel everywhere inside us. And how long might they stay in their search for opportunity?

Visit your liver, beneath your lungs, stomach, and heart. The repository of much of your blood like a train yard or a reservoir. Here, too, the virus may be present, and the liver's cells are busy with their process and manufacturing of your body's chemicals but are vigilant, too. Their function is an essential service, and distancing serves the whole. Filter your fluids, and suspect anyone who arrives carrying a key.

You are in your brain where special arteries are lined to create a blood-brain barrier. A natural Transportation Security Administration checking all that pass through, checking their luggage, checking their credentials.

There are not just one or two, there are billions. They are not here with an alternative, they are missionaries of a different god. Over the millennia they have brought foreign genes and exotic proteins from far off species, and some of what they bring we use, but they don't do it for our benefit. Like loan sharks, they exact a high price.

Feel your cells changing the locks on their doors and set your own terms. You can suffer a few, but not the multitudes. Like foreigners bearing the plague, make these travelers unwelcome. If you can't recognize them as different, then shut your doors to all foreigners.

The distancing is a different energy, a template, a way of our cells that deeply affects how we express ourselves, how we feel about ourselves. A much greater effect than our half-hearted, politically directed, social distancing. Your cells will not admit just any protein that wields a key. This is exclusion at a deep level.

Strip from your diet all toxins and bad habits. Eat only the cleanest food, drink the clearest water, breathe the purest air. Pay attention to the foods that help and those that slow you down. You don't want sugar, sweets, alcohol, or starch. Release your old habits and follow comfort and intuition from plants and protein.

Take a deep breath and check in with your body. Rely on your body. Return to your pulse and the sense of space within your body.

Translate this attitude to the cells of your body. Every sensation has intelligence. Be aggressively pure, cautious and protective at the level of your thoughts. These actions set an example for your organs, cells, and membranes. Your thoughts are much less voluntary than you assume; less of your free will and more of your body's inner wisdom. Responses motivated by the memory, perception, and needs of your tissues. Remain connected and listen deeply.

Remember this connection. Recall the voice of your body, a wise voice in a crowd. You will recognize this voice in everyday affairs, where it often goes unrecognized. Your inner wisdom has a resonance you will remember. The voice of your body is not the voice of your mind. Remember the grounded voice, it has an older memory and it wastes less time. It is not afraid, it is not distracted, it is strong and knows more than its age explains. It is a voice you hear and trust.

Return now to the thin level, the high altitude of intellect, logic, and constructions. So much that lacks foundation, and now you feel foundation, and you don't need to explain yourself, and you will not be swayed.

Enter an elevator that will take you back to your daily altitudes, See yourself rising from the microscopic. Scaling up from **one**, **two**, **three**, back to breathing from the outside looking in, **four**, **five**, **six**, looking around at the busy hub-bub of other people, **seven**, **eight**, **nine**. Take a breath. Inhale… exhale… And **ten**. The bell rings and you step out, eyes open, looking from the top down.

9 – Rethinking the Implausible

Of minds and molecules.

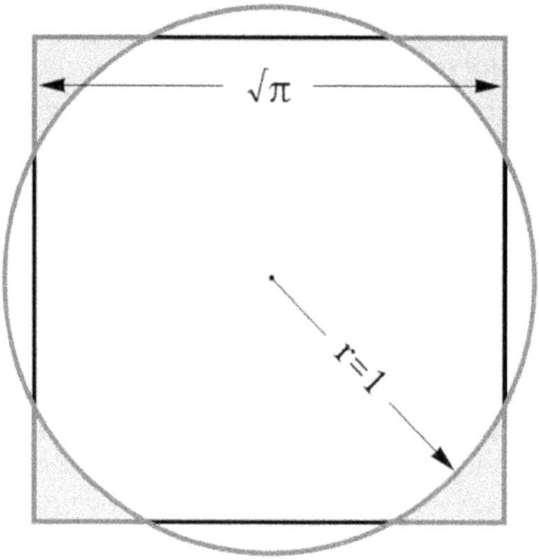

"Decades of research have established the general validity of the psycho-neuro-immunological response well beyond any reasonable doubt."
— **David Cheek and Ernest Rossi** (Cheek 1994, p. 202)

Movement of the Molecules

To say that a disease is of this organ or that organ presupposes a lot. It assumes that there's something special about the structure of the organ and the mechanism of the disease that links the two. This applies to tapeworms in the gut as well as cirrhosis of the liver, but it doesn't apply well to many viruses, and it certainly doesn't apply to SARS-CoV-2 whose mechanism is especially general. There really is no "disease" COVID-19, there is rather a broad state of biochemical disruptions.

Even this is too specific. Viruses are too simple to have a strategy because that would require them to negotiate changing events in order to maintain it. Instead, they have a varied toolkit with a good deal of redundancy and the ability to evolve quickly. Evolution is to a virus what thinking is to us. It takes longer–on the order of months—and it's not built on inference, it's built on feedback.

> "Humans describe the contest between host and virus as a war, but the virus is not at war. Our enemy has no agency; it does not develop 'strategies' for escaping our medicines or the activity of our immune systems… SARS-CoV-2 virus has no plan. It doesn't need one; absent a vaccine, the virus is here to stay. 'This is a pretty efficient pathogen,' Dr. Garry (microbiologist at Tulane University) said. 'It's very good at what it does.' "
>
> — **Alan Burdick** (Burdick, 2020), correspondent for the *New York Times.*

Evolution is a lot more scientific than the decisions we make based on conjecture. Evolution explores opportunities experimentally, and moves toward evidence-based results. Evolution never gets discouraged or depressed which gives viruses the ultimate Vulcan mentality: they just do what works in proportion to the result.

I'm not a virologist so I have to think in simple terms. I understand the virus in terms of three imperatives:

- find and enter an environment that provides the tools for its reproduction,
- use those tools to create copies of itself,
- find a way out and endure passage to the next reproductive environment.

Stopping the virus, from our point of view, can happen at any of these steps. Our efforts at isolation—both isolating ourselves from each other and isolating the virus from us—are attempts at denying the virus an environment in which to reproduce. That is a conceptually simple solution.

> "I usually picture it as an entity that comes into the cell and then it falls apart… It has to fall apart to build some mini-factories in the cell to reproduce itself, and has to come together as an entity at the end to infect other cells."
>
> — **Dr. Melanie Ott**, Director, Gladstone Institute of Virology

Our attempts to heal people suffering from a viral infection is a much more complicated problem as the damage is already done and the virus is accomplishing all three of its tasks. At that point, stopping one of the virus's main tasks will not make a person better, you need to stop all three.

This is only made more difficult when we say the virus is a disease that manifests specific symptoms because it doesn't. The problem of finding a cure is made more difficult by targeting the virus's symptoms rather than its causes.

The first major dysfunction caused by SARS-CoV-2 occurs at our membranes. The membranes first affected are the ones it first reaches, which is usually the upper respiratory tract. This becomes serious when the virus reaches the lower respiratory tract of people whose metabolism is already impaired.

For many people, notably the young and the healthy, the pulmonary system is not at risk and the virus will not do damage unless it gets beyond the respiratory tract. For these people, the gut is the first serious disruption. This usually resolves in a few days, but that doesn't mean the virus is gone, it's still in them and it's still looking for opportunity.

There are other points of vulnerability if the virus can get to them. If the virus makes it into the blood, then it can assail the circulatory system or any organ to which it can be delivered, including the skin and the brain.

Depending on the location, different systems will respond and with different symptoms. There will be different paths to recovery in each case. I would not be surprised if the virus could affect the joints if it could find a way to get there.

What's Going On?

> "We tend to think of the brain as being like a puppet master pulling strings, but in reality the brain is more like the symphony conductor bringing some things up, quieting other things down."
>
> — **H. Craig Heller**, PhD, in "The Molecules That Make Memory" (Brazil, 2014).

It helps to know a little of what the virus is doing. In truth, that's all we know: a little. We know the simple things like how we get infected, although the details depend on things we don't know. We don't know how well the virus survives out of the body, how it establishes itself in different tissues, or how some people prevent infection or minimize its effect. We know more about how the virus gets into cells, as that is advertised through the chemistry on the virus's surface. It gets into cells using its spike proteins that act as keys to the ACE2 receptor. That receptor bars entry to and is located on many different types of cells in our body.

We know less about how the virus marshals, or hijacks, our biochemistry to reproduce itself within our cell or insinuates itself into our DNA. It's here, we believe, that zinc plays a role in blocking viral reproduction, but there are many steps and many molecules involved.

We seem to know the least about how the virus reassembles itself, reconstituting itself from borrowed parts to be reborn by the millions as intact, cloned, and independent virions. This is the most complex and foreign step of the virus's three steps to reproduction. I have not heard any suggestions of how to stop the virus at this stage, while it's still within our cells.

Mind in Matter

> "Most of those studies found a positive association between the frequency of self-practice and optimized immune outcomes."
>
> — **Lemmy Schakel**, et al. (2019)

> "Those subjects who noted that they actually 'felt' something going on inside of their bodies were more likely to show changes in blood function as well. To what extent can people be trained prior to illness to be more aware of their bodies, even on a cellular level."
>
> — **Schneider, Smith, & Witcher** (1984).

Hypnosis and other forms of intentional healing, are not "mind over matter," they're mind in matter. They work through the mind's ability to have some effect on the health and metabolism of your organs. The results may seem miraculous, such as facilitating one's recovery from cancer, but this is not miraculous, it's simply the mind's ability to communicate with and help the body.

At the most conscious level, we can do things like eat, sleep, and exercise. At a chemical level we can to some extent intentionally release hormones associated with relaxation, confidence, determination, and positive intention. We can also have an effect on our body's electrical system.

Sadly, Western medicine knows next to nothing about the body's electrical system. Pharmacology sees electricity as something that makes drugs work. Neurology sees electricity as delivering information to a nervous system that does little more than release or inhibit chemicals. Clinical medicine knows electricity as little more than a means of burning tissue by delivering heat through laser and particle beams.

Acupuncture and Oriental Medicine, while not couched in electrical terms, are concerned with electrical systems when they talk about energizing a meridian or stimulating the body's chi. Physiotherapists and chiropractors are working with the nervous activation of tissues, and craniosacral therapists are sensing rhythms and currents in the body.

As I gain more experience and have more interaction with clinicians in other modalities I am beginning to understand why there is so little collective understanding: people who practice alternative modalities are not fully informed of what other practitioners do. Everyone speaks a specialized language.

I have been interested in bio-electrical systems since I accidentally met Robert O. Becker, MD, in the 1980s, before he wrote the book *The Body Electric: Electromagnetism And The Foundation Of Life*. It was another 20 years before I met Frank Echenhofer, who conducted the early research on the brainwaves of Buddhist monks. After that, I started my own practice with brainwaves as a neurofeedback therapist. This led to my tinkering with other electrical-based approaches such as Direct Cranial Stimulation, Infrared Light Therapy, and others, many of which have matured into fields of their own.

There are few physicists involved in medical technology, so few practitioners understand their tools in a way that satisfies me. The engineers understand how they work, and the clinicians know how to use them, but no one seems to care why they work. It's really a case of people being uninterested in those questions which they don't have the tools to answer.

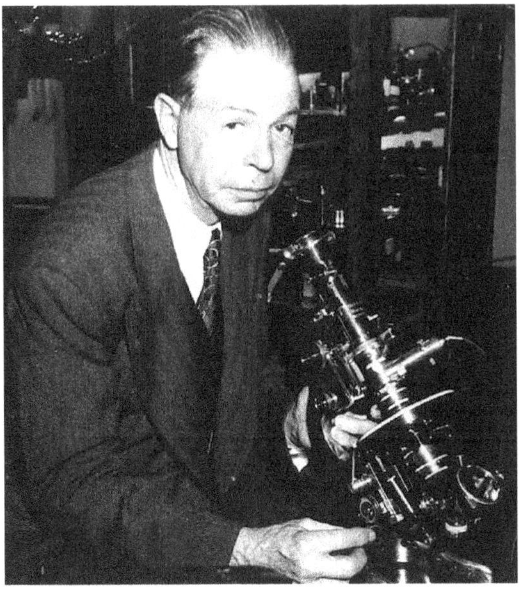

Royal Raymond Rife

Fields and Feelings

In the 1920s and 1930s Royal Rife, an inventor, engineer, and professional microscopist living in Southern California, developed some of the first field-effect microscopes. His machines achieved unheard of magnifications using oscillating, polarized light. Rife claimed viruses and bacteria would fluoresce, and he could both see and perform experiments on them *in vivo*, something that cannot be done with viruses, today (Walker, 2020).

It has since been pointed out by a well-meaning microscopist that Rife's claim of 30,000x resolution was physically impossible with a visible-light microscope (Hudson-Smith, 2017), but this is narrow-minded and it's wrong. Rife was using ultraviolet light that allows finer resolution than visible light, and, more importantly, he was using an oscillating field that made his subject fluoresce.

> "At various declinations of the refracted and polarized ray normally invisible bodies would become visible in a color peculiar to their structure or chemical make-up."
>
> — **Peter Walker**, referring to Rife's observations (Walker, 2020).

> "When that portion of the spectrum is reached in which both the organism and the color band vibrate in exact accord, one with the other, a definite characteristic spectrum is emitted by the organism."
>
> — **The Smithsonian Report**, describing how others understood Rife's result (Skidel & Winter, 1945).

> "In the 1990s, the potential for overcoming the diffraction barrier was realized, and microscopy concepts were defined that now resolve fluorescent features down to molecular dimensions."
>
> — **Sahl, Schönle, & Hell** (2019), in "Fluorescence Microscopy with Nanometer Resolution," describing what was re-discovered and explained 70 years after Rife.

Rife was performing a kind of spectroscopy of the resonant structures of living organisms—what he referred to as their refraction properties. By watching bacteria and viruses in their living state, Rife said that he could observe the effect of impinging electrical waves. He said he could tune these waves to the pathogen's resonant frequencies, and kill them. For this purpose, he built "ray machines" that focused broadband, low-frequency electrical radiation. He claimed near-perfect success in curing cancers, and, apparently, had clinical data to back this up.

Sixty years after Rife, others built similar fluorescent-field microscopes with even greater resolution. But we don't know what Rife saw since his notes were lost and his instruments destroyed. One might think that his claims of curing cancers, which were dismissed, would be revisited, but they have not been.

Profits and Progress

We may never know if Rife's cure for disease was real or practical. But we do know other claims of importance have been badgered, bludgeoned, burned, and bamboozled into submission for financial gain. And while you may have faith in the integrity of your doctor, you should not have faith in the medical industry because—like all cartels—it must put profits first (Davis, 2007). This is not an option, it's the law: corporations are legally obliged to put shareholder profits above all else. Because of this, industries are suspicious of innovation.

For example, we all now know of the dangers of nicotine and lead, but few of us know the claim that lead-containing products were poisoning us was fought tooth and nail by the industries that profited from it (Kitman, 2000). It took Clair Patterson, an exceptional scientist, a lifetime to substantiate the observations that resulted in eliminating levels of lead from our bodies which, by the late 20th-century, were 100 times their historical levels (Reilly, 2017).

Patterson was obstructed by the oil industry and its many associates at every turn. In spite of his being an odd personality, he prevailed because he preserved his institutional protection, was a consummate researcher, and had broad academic support. In contrast, Rife was a loner whose narrow base of support was chipped away.

Rife's "to hell with what other people think, I know what I see" attitude is typical of intuitive engineers. An intuitive engineer may seem like an oxymoron, but it is the foundation of genius. You can witness this yourself in two of my mentors, Charles Townes and Jerry Lettvin, whose interviews I recorded in my book *The Learning Project* (Stoller, 2019c). Townes and Lettvin achieved the impossible—producing monochromatic light and measuring signals from a single axon—and, in doing so, revolutionized their fields of physics and neurophysiology.

Not Completely Forgotten

At first, Rife's work was celebrated. Throughout the 1930s he had widespread success in clinics and laboratories, but it was too soon for the business of medicine. Energy medicine had no footing; commercial interests became involved. Subsequent legal battles led to his machines being confiscated, two laboratories burned under suspicious circumstances, his notes lost, and all details of his work eventually forgotten. It's a sad story that illustrates that medicine is not a science, and research follows commercial interests.

Now, long after his death in 1971, observations similar to Rife's have emerged (Yamazaki, 2020; Vadalà et al., 2016). There are clinics in Europe and one in Arizona that openly offer Rife-related therapy.

You can use what today is called a Rife Machine—which only remotely reflects what Rife developed. The electrical radiation generated by these machines is neither monochromatic nor thermal. It is low frequency, broadband, and broadly harmonic in its spectra. I have not seen any actual spectral measurements, but from the simple design of the machine, I can see that the spectra it generates are complex.

"Rifing" stimulates one's tissues. It can result in tingling, heating, irritation, and even inflammation. It can also create fatigue, headaches, and flu-like symptoms. The results resemble what one feels after an acupuncture session.

I must caution you: Rife machines are entirely unapproved for medical use in the US. No one would think of applying to the FDA for certification because there is no accepted theory behind them, no accepted clinical direction about how to use them, no funding for them, and they are considered pseudo-science. Of course, all new science can be called "pseudo-science" until it's accepted science. I'm not concerned with using the Rife machine here. I mention it only because it suggests something about hypnosis and energy medicine.

Naturally, I have a Rife machine, or what passes as one. Every few years I set it up and irradiate myself looking for efficacious frequencies. The Rife machine generates sensations in me I otherwise do not have. Just as with acupuncture, I gain a feeling of warmth and invigoration, and I can work with these feelings using my imagination. What's more important, once I've had these feelings, I can often regain them using my imagination alone. That takes us back to hypnosis.

I don't know how to use my mind to make chemical changes within my cells, but I can use my mind to change how my tissues feel if I can feel those tissues. When I change how my tissues feel I'm changing something in my cells, perhaps not directly but certainly indirectly, in terms of what I'm doing to those cells.

The key is to be able to change feelings in your tissues. If you have no feeling, then there's nothing you can change. But once you have some feeling, then you can shape, expand, and even speak to it. It's on this basis that I offer my next induction, *Mind and Molecules*.

"The immune system may be considered a cellular extension of the brain, a 'mobile sensory organ.' "

— **R. Zachariae, et al.** (1990), in "Effect of Psychological Intervention in the Form of Relaxation and Guided Imagery on Cellular Immune Normal Healthy Subjects."

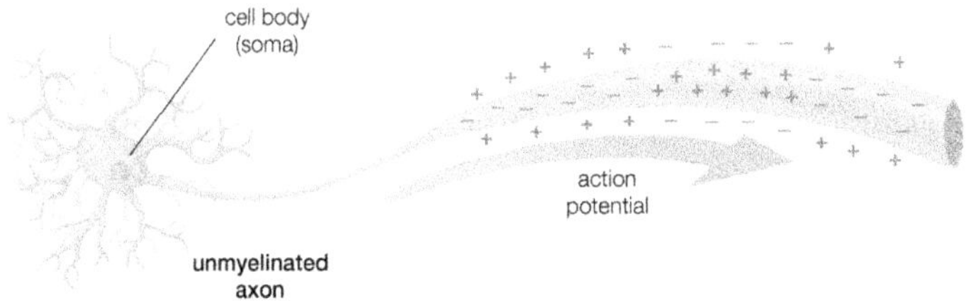

Hypnotic Session 8

Mind and Molecules audio file at:
https://www.mindstrengthbalance.com/covid19-illness-illumination/

Mind and Molecules

Mind and Molecules is a hypnotic induction that requires your full attention. Do not listen to this hypnotic visualization if you are driving a car, operating machinery, or doing anything that requires your attention.

Like all of my inductions, *Mind and Molecules* involves both what I believe will help you, and what I have experienced as helpful. *Mind and Molecules* involves creating or amplifying feelings, and then enlarging and enlivening those feelings.

You cannot fail at this, but you can do less or more according to the measure of your engagement. The more deeply you engage, the larger and more powerful an experience you'll create. The whole premise rests on the connection between your mind's experience and your body's response. Deeper is better, and the only thing down there is you.

I ask for your wordless experience, for you to experience sensations in your body wordlessly. The words I use feel like a thin whitewash over the printed page of your mind's talk, moving back and forth, layering coat after coat. I replace your words with my words, and your words with my words. And I do that because it's not the words I want—I don't want words at all—I want no words, but our minds are word addicts.

Words are like oil to an engine, they must be there even when idling otherwise your mind starts to strain. It's true that by meditating you can experience short bursts of wordlessness, but they're short. The only way to really escape the word trap is to escape the mind, and where you go when you do this is unclear. Most likely you will either go into your body or into an uncontained experience.

Both alternatives are valuable, both are natural, and both are ever-present, you are just less aware of them, or not aware of them at all. They are states that lie between your states of awareness and that's OK. They can operate in the background. These states take care of your body automatically. They emerge to inspire and guide you when you need them.

If you want to move forward with greater assurance, or if you need to find greater strength, or health, or clarity, or purpose, then you must set off to find these transition states willfully and—it must be said—at some risk. Disruption is always a risk, but if your health, spirit, or direction is already disrupted, then there is no choice.

I say this to remind you that depth is important. Depth of experience is essential. What you get out of all thinking—this experience included—rests on how much attention you focus on it, focus on this and nothing else.

Find a comfortable position lying down. Let the muscles of your chest and torso relax without any need to hold your head up or body upright. We are not aware of the actions of our muscles to keep us upright, but our muscles must be attentive in order to keep us so. I want to take your attention on these muscles elsewhere, along with all the nerves and sensations they rely on. Relax and loosen all the muscles in your shoulders, neck, and torso.

Close your eyes, or dim your eyes, and put your attention on the front of your body. I'd like you to focus on an area I'll call your breast but I don't mean "breasts," I mean that area below your chin and above your solar plexus. That thin, flat, bony area below your collar bone that we call your breastplate.

This is an area we don't speak much about but we very much put it forward. We don't beat it like an ape or display it like a robin, but there remains something powerful about it. It's what we bare to show our bravery, what we offer to represent ourselves in courage and sacrifice. What we offer in proximity and relax in trust.

Men inflate their breasts to increase their presence. Women adorn theirs with pendants and jewelry. The breastplate is a part of our anatomy involved with movement and transit: our aorta, esophagus, and our windpipe. From it we project our voice. The breastplate is part of our thorax, within it are found our heart and lungs, and it's a very mortal area.

I have described this area, and I'd like you to sense the feeling beyond this description, beyond simply the place in your body. This area from which love emanates and in which we feel the hole of heartbreak. It is vulnerable and central. It does not speak and our voice does not come from it, but it is an emotional center, a center of strength. If there was a place where "The Force" resides, it's here.

Leave this area now and let relaxation start in your limbs. Feel the relaxation in your hands and feet, and relax your neck and head. If you were star-shaped, then these would be your points: hands, feet, and head. Imagine that these points radiate like a star, and they burn like beacons all the time, ready to act or think or move, all places in the thought or act of movement. Your extremities have an incessant sense of activity and preparedness.

Feel a sense of vibrancy in your hands, a high frequency, a rapid rhythm, as if they're always wound up and ready to move at the slightest inclination. Turn that frequency down and make your hands feel more relaxed, warmer, heavier, as if connected with fibers or threads to the earth. Feel the desire to relax and release your hands from your mind's incessant need to demonstrate or gesture.

Feel your hands so relaxed that they go off-line, as if they're down for maintenance, and they won't move. No matter what your authority, no matter how casual your expectation, your hands won't move because they're warm, and comfortable, and quiet, like someone tucked into a warm bed, your hands are resting.

Now feel your feet. They follow a slower rhythm. They don't reach for things or gesticulate, but they do stretch and they have a mind to walk. They like to walk, they like to move in alternation. As they are bilateral they integrate your awareness.

They are the first on the checklist of moving forward, making progress, and putting things into position. They connect us and we feel wonderful when they're comfortable. They have a slower rhythm but also a more noticeable rhythm, to be rubbed, soothed, or cushioned. They too have a vibrating energy, and you can turn that up and turn it down simply by focusing your attention.

Focus your attention on your feet. Mentally relax those bones and muscles that are always packed and ready to come to your service. Your arches, your heels, the sides of your feet, the balls of your feet, and your toes. Wrap them in a ball of warm red light and let them get warmer, slower, and heavier. Feeling rested and connected.

Feel the energy in your feet growing, glowing, and moving a consciousness up your calves and through your knees, as if they were beneath a heavy blanket and you can feel them getting warmer and heavier, and soon you have the feeling that they won't move, they don't want to move, and that they can silently refuse your mind's commands and they rest, being comfortable and grounded.

This energy in your feet and this energy in your hands—an almost palpable kind of energy that is like an internal sensation, not felt on the skin but along the bones. It moves inward engulfing your wrists and ankles causing a deeper kind of rest when it reaches your knees and elbows. The bones relax, and their joints relax, and you feel further rooted to the spot as now both your knees and elbows refuse to move. They don't want to move; they're comfortable, resting, and relaxed.

Imagine that your hands and feet are charging, like plugs. They are connected to the ground and conduct an earth current that provides a slow and growing stream of power. Let those connections settle, and change.

Bring your attention to your head. Imagine you wanted to gain a clarity that centered your thoughts. Something that settled your mind. Imagine the kind of calm, settled connection that you can feel in your hands and feet as something that can recharge your mind. Imagine this comes from the sky, the clouds, the air, or the trees, not as a lightning bolt but as a slower, crackling current.

The sky does have a charge and currents do move through the air and you hear them as static on the radio. The air is a poor conductor so this charge is slow. Let it recharge you, slowly, like a charger charges a battery, not a surge but a steady flow, a trickle charge.

What would this feel like in your mind? Would it require you to be asleep, detached, or resting? Release the staccato of words and ideas. Can you feel the charge if you pace your breath and let your thoughts flow as smooth perception?

Turn down the spigot of words and thoughts. Turn it off completely if you can, but if you can't then let it drip, an irrigation of words to complement the slow drip of electrical charge fortifying your head and skull, down through your neck and into your body. A bone consciousness, a relaxed container, patching a bucket's holes while your thoughts swim like fish inside it.

Spend this moment resting in that state of recharging: your hands and feet are warm. They conduct a current from your limbs into your body. Your head is recharging and your thoughts wander in circles or settle to the bottom of the tank while the filters flush and new molecules fill the cracks in your consciousness.

Take a breath, breathing from that central core to which your appendages connect, so that on the inhale you feel yourself pulling in not only air but energy. Energy from the earth through your limbs and from the sky through your head.

If you're in daylight, outdoors, or under an open sky, then let your arms, hands, and fingers act like antennas, lightning rods, the vanes of windmills collecting energy from the air, currents, sunlight, and movement.

This energy comes into you subtly, like charge or chi or heat or sound, all moving toward your center, toward your solar plexus, your torso, your thorax, your breast. Moving into and around your heart and lungs to become incorporated in your circulation, charging your blood, and feeding your tissues.

Return now to the front of you, the breast, the window of your heart, and feel these energies dancing beneath the surface of your skin. Focus on this part of your body and imagine it is a charging plate, and from it your aura bubbles like a spring.

Feel a movement just on your skin like little waves spreading across a puddle, pushed by the wind. Feel this building, swelling, fortifying your breast from side to side, from the muscles across your chest, to those that wrap around your ribs, to the muscles layered in alternation across your back.

This is expansion and energy. You are a battery and this is your charge. It swells and powers and fills its container. It is an energy for healing, recovery, and action. You use it for rebuilding, thought, or movement.

Every day when you connect, and every night when you sleep, you bring these energies in and recharge like a battery, a power plant, a core. You see the meter on your battery pack: five, thick green bars that pulse as you build them up.

First there's **one**: a single glowing bar. It grows to **two**, and then rises to **three**, now **four** pulsing, vibrant bars. Now at **five** bars, and you have gained full power.

Your body relies on this charge, it powers your many parts: organs, cells, membranes, muscles, ions, chemicals, molecules. It powers movement and communication, creation and destruction, conversion of forms, elimination of waste, repair and reassembly. Insight, inspiration, anger, and love.

Imagine that you can feel this charge as you felt it in your hands and feet, and you can feel it as energy in your mind. Push this energy into your tissues, membranes, and molecules. Draining like a heartbeat, pushed out of your core, your battery, distributed to all parts within you:

Five, channeling along your bones.

Four, filling tissues like filling a lake.

Three, charging your separate organs.

Two, cleansing pathways, unobstructed.

And **one** inhale… and exhale...

Throughout your breast you feel this energy as an expanse, sometimes quiet and other times vibrant. You might or might not feel it now, you might feel it at other times: in the afternoon, late at night, or upon waking in the night.

Whenever you feel energized, or whenever you need energy, you can stop and focus, measure and monitor this level of energy. Some days it's high, others it's low, and your moods ride it like a cork on water. It flows out from your heart and back in through your hands and feet:

One, tingling in your fingers.

Two, coming in through your feet.

Three, rising up through your arms.

Four, rising past your knees and thighs.

And **five**, filling your torso, a full container.

Broadcast this energy throughout your body, especially into those areas that feel too quiet, need the most healing, or feel low-energy. Cells or tissues that need energy and you can minister to them as your soldiers.

Processes need reinforcements. It's not a war but it is a struggle. Channels open within your body to take, move, channel, and transport these energies into those tissues to be revitalized. The long march of health to the wide horizon of longevity.

Five, into your lungs.

Four, into your bloodstream.

Three, into your gut and digestion.

Two, up into your brain for calm and clarity.

One, inhale into your heart center… and exhale...

At times this energy may feel low, like water draining from a shallow pool, and other times it's overflowing. Bring it in with your inhale, settling yourself into a receptive place. Pull this energy in from your hands and feet, into the center of yourself, through a calm and focused mind.

One, open and accepting.

Two, receiving and welcoming.

Three, grateful and attentive.

Four, aware of the work of others.

Five, connected with a simple purpose.

Relax and drift. Calm in service to your own needs, the higher good of those around you. There is a cycle of filling and emptying, and that's OK, everything moves in cycles. You may feel tired at one moment and energized at another, and that's OK.

Imagine a wide flat battery behind your breast-plate. It's a power source, like lithium ion or hydrogen fuel. It takes time to charge or recharge, but it can hold its charge, and you can find the sources to charge it in the natural world around you.

And when you charge it to whatever level is comfortable, it may activate you like a cup of coffee, or it may pacify you, like a full meal. Either way you can move with it, feel the cycle of it, recognize your need to support it, be in synchrony with it.

Returning now to feeling your whole body as one, as some super-modern, complex instrument; a self-generating power station moving through space, gathering energy from all resources, collecting, retaining, distributing, resting, and recharging.

Keep that sense of awareness in your breast-plate, as if your mind has a meter. Whenever you need to manage your day and your life, you only need to consult this meter in your mind to know if you have enough energy or if you need more. It is your gas gauge, fuel gauge, and battery meter. It is your oxygen meter, your air tank, altimeter, and your pressure gauge.

Come back now, keeping that feeling of managing power from the center of your star, the navigator of your body, the builder of your health. Coming back to energize the star, counting to five, starting at the center.

> **One**, the core, the power, the pile. The central power station that is your body.
>
> **Two,** for the symmetry of your body, the left and the right. Inhale… exhale…
>
> **Three**, as you energize the core, the organs around it, your bones and skin.
>
> **Four**, your arms and legs, fastening you to the earth and managing what's in your grasp.
>
> And **five**, you light up like a star, connected and connecting your feet to the ground.

Your hands to what you touch, and your head to what you see, hear, and say. Take a breath. Inhale… exhale… and settle back into calmness. Back to your body and mind.

---

10 – Viral Fatigue

When the virus does not leave your body.

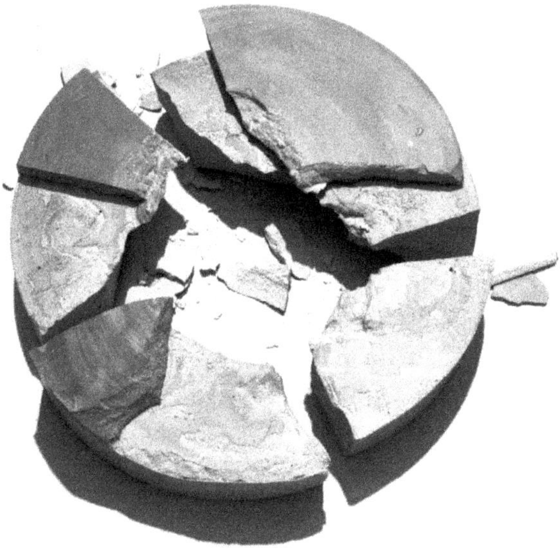

"When you have exhausted all possibilities, remember this: you haven't."
— **Thomas Edison**

Short-Sighted

When COVID-19 first appeared all attention was on the fear of death and the lack of immunity. In general, it seems, attention is focused on the sensational. This is a bad way to approach a risky situation. Only slowly has attention turned to remaining healthy and understanding transmission.

The pandemic has progressed much as epidemiologists predicted. However, the symptoms are not as clear as originally thought. Those at risk are more specific in their vulnerabilities, and the virus's transmission is more subtle. Because of these factors—which are not only different from what was presumed but have changed over time—the mortality rate is lower than was originally feared, though still five to ten times higher than influenza.

Now, three months into the official pandemic, measuring from March 11th when the WHO assigned that designation—and three months after COVID-19 first appeared—the public understanding is still thin and the political discussions shallow. This is in spite of plenty of expertise and experience.

We know the virus is still present and that widespread infection will reappear once the population again begins to intermingle. We know we need to monitor infection levels to navigate the near-term, and that requires widespread testing. In spite of this, little testing is being done. As a result, we can expect there will be a resurgence of infection which could exceed initial levels, judging from past pandemics. This is only one of many issues not part of the political dialog.

Discussions of cures, treatments, and preventatives—including the prospect of vaccination—erupt daily in the mainstream press. These come to a head, spill dire warnings or hopeful promises, and then fade away. In spite of this, there has been no interest in becoming educated in these issues. The vaccine/anti-vaccine diatribe remains sophomoric, issues pertaining to strengthening immunity remain anecdotal, and treatments are no better understood than the symptoms of the illness, which are widely varied.

Post-Infection

Even less discussed is what happens after one gets COVID-19. There seems to be a general and ignorant avoidance of the inconvenient fact that just as COVID-19 is not a particular illness—it can and often does affect multiple systems in different ways—it is not something that one simply "recovers" from.

In this, SARS-CoV-2 is not that unique. Viral afflictions, in general, are not diseases, they are infections, and this one seems particularly complex. One of the consequences of many viral infections—and we can presume this will be a consequence of SARS-CoV-2—is something called Post Viral Fatigue Syndrome, or PVFS.

It's not clear what PVFS is, but it seems to develop as a consequence of many viral illnesses. Its symptom is similar to CFS, Chronic Fatigue Syndrome, characterized by extreme and long-lasting fatigue. In spite of the similarity in name and symptoms, CFS has a method for diagnosis, though it is in dispute, while PVFS does not. The diagnosis is said to involve extensive tests and a medical history which makes for a complicated but not necessarily accurate process. Suffice it to say that neither PVFS nor CFS are well understood.

It's estimated that 20% of those who recover from serious viral illnesses experience some form of PVFS, but PVFS often goes undiagnosed. Many of us have experienced a slow recovery from an illness and it's not clear whether or not this is to be expected with COVID-19. Nor is it clear when a recovery is very slow, whether it is a recovery from the original illness, or a continuation of it. This seems to be especially true with COVID-19 whose infection causes enduring symptoms.

My first suspected symptoms of COVID-19 were mild. They appeared on March 17th and lasted for five days. Because I'd already had what I believed to be the seasonal flu, and because these symptoms were unusual, I considered COVID-19 a likely cause. Two weeks later I had a serious gastrointestinal infection that developed within hours, affected my whole G.I. tract, and disappeared 48 hours later. This also fit the COVID-19 profile.

Seven weeks have now past since the G.I. infection and my night sweats, lassitude, and malaise have reoccured on a regular schedule. In addition, I find myself drawn to carbohydrates and proteins, and I am now experienced a newfound difficulty with sugar and egg products.

Fatigue is Common

In a proposed study on COVID-19 I read:

> "Chronic fatigue is the most common and debilitating symptom in intensive care unit (ICU) survivors. Indeed, it has been widely reported that patients who stayed in ICU for prolonged periods report a feeling of tiredness for months to years after ICU discharge. This symptom seems particularly pronounced in Covid-19 patients and may affect their quality of life by decreasing their capacity to perform simple tasks of daily life."
>
> — from "Chronic Fatigue Etiology and Recovery in Covid-19 Patients: the Role of Fatigability (FatCovid-19)," (NIH, 2020).

While I have not been hospitalized, it is not the hospitalization that causes the disturbance. I suspect my gut flora has been disturbed by the infection. Taking a low dose of probiotics, which seemed to have an initial positive effect, was not restoring my vitality. This was when I researched post-viral syndromes and found that CFS appears to have a substantial relationship to gut health, and that efforts to repopulate the gut biota had long-term success in 30 - 50% of diagnosed cases (Roman et al., 2018; Venturini et al., 2019).

> "While most people with post-infection fatigue will improve and return to normal health, good management during the very early stage is an important factor in trying to help any natural recovery process take place. And patient evidence also indicates that good initial management of post-infection fatigue lessens the chances of this turning into an ME/CFS-like illness."
>
> — **Dr Charles Shepherd** (Shepherd, 2020), *ME Association.*

The Gut

The gut is an essential part of your immune system. It's where your leukocytes get their chemical education. Your blood is both the source of your body's nutrition and the vehicle for your immune defense and both functions are largely empowered in your gut. For more detail, read the article, "Why Gut Bacteria are Essential for a Healthy Immune System," (Medicalxpress, 2018).

Taking matters into my own hands, and having success with past fasts, I decided to repopulate my G.I. tract. Because I was experiencing difficulty with sugar, which is implicated with flair-ups of gut candida and because of other contra-indications against sugars such as found in most juice, I limited myself to water, vitamins, and mild laxatives for the duration of a 3-day fast.

Each day I mixed filtered water with a package of Emergen-C powder along with a multivitamin. Emergen-C provides 1-gram of vitamin C (the recommended daily allowance (RDA) is 0.1 grams) along with a minor dose of additional vitamins.

I also took 2,000 UIs of vitamin D (twice the RDA), 100 mg of zinc (ten times the RDA for zinc), and 500 mg of quercetin—a bioflavonoid for which there is no RDA, but this was half the typical dose.

With this, I consumed over the course of each day: two 8 oz glasses of water mixed with Metamucil (psyllium husks), several cups of senna leaf tea (a laxative), two cups of organic prune juice—which provided quite a bit of natural sugar—and as much water as I could, which I mixed with a pinch of salt.

On the first day I felt weak and slept for several hours in the afternoon. On the second day my energy stabilized and I went for a 2-hour walk. I ended the third day feeling well-slept and took a 90-minute hike up a 200-meter hill.

I was never hungry over the course of the fast, but after three days I planned to break the fast by reintroducing first probiotics in capsule form, which consists of a spectrum of bioflora. I then ate prebiotics—roughage, which is food for the probiotics—and finally food. It's important to break a fast carefully.

Before bed on the third day, I mixed my first dose of probiotic powder with a few tablespoons of sauerkraut, a cup of water, and a few tablespoons of yogurt whey. I drank two cups of water through the night and in the morning of the fourth day took my second dose of probiotics with similar hydration.

A few hours later I ate my first meal: a large plate of well-cooked shredded cabbage and carrot. I continued a diet of cooked, low sugar, unspiced, low fat, high-roughage foods and herbal teas until returning to my normal, carnivorous, healthy diet by the fifth day.

Since the point of this effort was to repopulate my digestive tract, I was particularly interested in the contents of the many different probiotic capsules available, and in comparing them to what were used in variously reported investigations.

Probiotics

We're currently experiencing a revolution in understanding the huge effect our gut health has on our mind, body, and levels of performance. While we still cannot establish direct causation between individual gut bacteria and our response to them, we're now finding ways to compare the profiles of people's gut bacteria with groups of people distinguished by their mental and physical characteristics (Ferry, 2018).

An article in *The Journal of Food and Drug Analysis* says:

"Research in probiotics has progressed considerably in the past two decades and significant advances have been made in the selection and characterization of specific probiotic cultures along with substantial health benefits upon consumption."

— **Rout Kerry, et al.** (Kerry et al., 2018) "Benefaction of probiotics for human health: A review."

In spite of this, I found no useful recommendations for what specific probiotic cultures to use in repopulating my digestive tract. Instead, I followed the general suggestions provided by Carol Wolf in her report "Did Probiotics Cure My Chronic Fatigue Syndrome?" (Wolf, 2016).

Finding herself in the same situation as me, she suggests using as high a bacterial count as one can tolerate, and the widest range of different bacteria that one can find. Not feeling the need to go overboard, as she admitted that she had, I settled on taking 300 billion bacteria per day, spread out through the day, which is roughly three times the maximum recommended amount. The chance of anything like an overdose seemed remote for me, and its consequence of irritation or diarrhea could be easily countered by lowering the dose.

Probiotics can trigger adverse reactions in immune-compromised individuals, so before you experiment with them do some research. If you have not taken them before and you'd like to, then start slowly. See the article, "Can You Overdose on Probiotics?" (Labdoor, 2017).

Be aware the gut bacteria of men and women differ significantly. It's important to add the right bacteria. For more information see Scott Anderson's "Sex and the Microbiome," at *Psychology Today*, (Anderson, 2020).

I compared the bacterial ingredients in most of the wide-spectrum probiotics —which I reviewed in the refrigerated section of my local Whole Foods store— to a half dozen alternatives listed on the VitaCost.com website. I found many of them contained the same bacteria. I settled on two, broad-spectrum probiotic capsules, a 90 billion Colony Forming Units (CFU), a 23-strain product sold by New Roots and labeled "Colon Care Probiotics," and a 100 billion CFU, 34-strain product by Garden of Life labeled "Ultimate Care."

I could have purchased any of the various other products, but found these gave me the largest number and the widest variety of bacteria for the lowest prices. The first provided 15 strains of Lactobacillus, 7 strains of Bifidobacterium, and one strain of Streptococcus. The second, 14 of Lactobacillus, 4 of Bifidobacterium, 1 of Streptococcus, 3 of Lactococcus, 4 of Leuconostoc, 4 of Saccharomyces, plus a few others. Without any guidance—

and I found no guidance—one can only aim for variety and hope that more is better.

Your gut is deeply involved in the health of your immune system, and unbalanced gut biota generate a wide variety of negative health conditions. In addition, gut health affects your moods, which you can experience as wide mood swings while fasting.

If you take probiotics you may notice they also precipitate mood swings. This should really catch your attention: if you can change your state of mind by adding live bacteria to your gut, just where is your state of mind located? I don't take this question lightly, and I don't think you should, either. For more information see Peter Bongiorno's, "The Gut Microbiome, Anxiety and Depression: 6 Steps to Take, How balancing your intestinal bugs brings balanced mood," in *Psychology Today* (Bongiorno, 2014).

It's too early to judge the success of my effort to rebalance my gut. Some people report rapid improvement, but the research studies span months of probiotic treatment. In general, changing one's gut biota takes months. My effort may take weeks or months to settle. So far, however, after only a few days, I'm feeling better. The night sweats are tapering off, but I'm still low on energy.

Hypnosis and the Gut

You will not be surprised that I propose to use hypnosis to address gut conditions since I've used it to address everything else. You may be surprised that psychological methods have been tested in this context and demonstrated a robust, positive effect.

> "Cognitive-behavioral therapy (CBT) has been tested most rigorously in multiple randomized controlled trials and consistently demonstrates significant and durable effects on Irritable Bowel Syndrome (IBS) symptoms and quality of life… Despite the well-documented advantages of CBT for IBS, it has been poorly disseminated and few patients have access to this treatment… the American Gastroenterological Association recommends psychological interventions for patients with moderate-to severe IBS."
>
> — **Sarah Kinsinger** (Kinsinger, 2017), "Cognitive-behavioral therapy for patients with irritable bowel syndrome: Current insights."

Irritable Bowel Syndrome is not Chronic Fatigue Syndrome, and the positive results obtained for the therapy of one don't imply similar results will ensue in a similar treatment of the other. On the other hand, both IBS and CFS are believed to have their origin partly, or largely, in the balance of gut biota.

What remains entirely unclear is whether addressing a person's psychology affects their gut directly or indirectly. That is, while we know they're connected, does working with the mind address the gut or the brain? Perhaps this is not a valid question; perhaps the two are so deeply intertwined that there is no point in trying to separate them.

On that basis, I offer the piece *The Harmony of the Microbes*, which is a guided visualization toward a balanced gut ecosystem. It approaches the balancing of one's gut from two directions: imagining an ego-centered sense of relief, and imagining a microbe-centered sense of harmony.

On the one hand, what you know about your gut is largely limited to what you feel. When your gut is well-balanced you feel control, balance, strength, and comfort. Projecting those feelings into your gut is your mind's way of entraining gut health.

On the other hand, we can imagine what it might feel like to inhabit a strong and balanced gut. That is, we can imagine what strength and balance might mean to a microbe who lives in your intestines. It may well be hopeless to try to "speak microbe," or to hope this image is accurate, but regardless of whether or not our imagination is accurate, it can still have an effect.

We already know our mind controls some elements of our gut environment, so we know we can affect it. Our mind creates the chemicals that affect our gut, and the microbes in our gut use these chemicals to communicate. There are many portals of communication; there is communication to the gut, and there is feedback from it.

In any fully interlinked system, it does not matter to which "link" you speak as each link affects the others. It is in this sense that the question, "Can one's psychology affect the gut biota?" is the wrong question. We know it can. The correct question is, how much can we accomplish.

Down the Final Stretch

After four months of feeling ill or under the weather, I'm starting to recover from Sars-Cov-2. My energy levels are growing and lassitude is shrinking. My nighttime bouts of dehydration—which wake me up every two hours to drink two cups of water and which used to be nightly—are now two weeks apart.

I'm running on intuition. I'm avoiding refined sugars and finding roughage suits my digestion. My need for protein has tapered off and my stomach feels stronger.

Exercise feels important and it's leaving me less fatigued. The immune system requires exercise—that's what pumps its fluids—so I'm out for walks of varying lengths every day. Sleep is always essential and I try to get plenty of it. I've even started moving toward a more diurnal sleep and waking cycle.

I'm weaning myself off of probiotics and returning to restorative herbals: dandelion root tea—a traditional herbal for liver and digestive support—powdered turmeric in everything—an anti-inflammatory, antioxidant, and mood enhancer—and a return to my elderberry decoction added to black tea. It seems my gut is returning to normal.

Social distancing, quarantine, movement restrictions, and border closures remain, but I am looking forward getting out for some long walks in the mountains. Hopefully, the virus and its symptoms are leaving my system after four months. I may be average; for others, it's taking longer (Yong, 2020).

Hypnotic Session 9

The Harmony of the Microbes audio file at:
https://www.mindstrengthbalance.com/covid19-illness-illumination/

The Harmony of the Microbes

The Harmony of the Microbes is a hypnotic induction that requires your full attention. Do not listen to this hypnotic visualization if you are driving a car, operating machinery, or doing anything that requires your attention.

This guided visualization speaks to the feelings in your gut, and speaks to your gut as a consciousness that can hear you. Begin by relaxing your mind and opening yourself to the idea that part of your personality exists in your gut. Let's explore what this means.

Find a relaxed position and consider the sound of my voice. My voice comes from some device, in which it has been reduced, it is broadcast as soundless vibrations, and it is converted back into a voice inside your head. This is not my voice, these are my ideas, but it is your voice. You are speaking my ideas.

If this sounds unsanitary, let me reassure you that my voice has been sterilized. My ideas may confuse you, but you will understand those that hold meaning for you. You are listening to energy, and you are converting this into thoughts. And from somewhere in your mind you are hearing words—most likely it is in your head. Relax that sense of location and allow yourself to hear me from other places in your body.

Imagine that you exist in your head, and all the voices you hear reside there. Your head is not an echo chamber, it's more like a pudding and the words you hear are its flavor, and this flavor is constantly changing. It changes in waves that pass through it. Let words be waves in this pudding and the thoughts they create be firm areas, while there is uncertainty in the softer places.

Take a breath, inhale… and exhale… and let these ideas coalesce into form as I count from five to one.

> Start at **five** and hear the word "relax," and do that into a smooth texture. A star with five points. Your breath is calm.
>
> Now at **four**. A square with four corners, and there is a skin to the idea that you are calm with this container, feeling yourself as a body.
>
> Three, the **three** points of a triangle with clarity, strength, and balance. A sense of center from which you are and see things.
>
> **Two**, a balance beam: two sides, two views, two phases, two feelings, two actions, the inhale… the exhale…
>
> And **one**, the self, the whole, the sense of being you. A sphere, a circle, the pointlessness of having any corners at all.

You are now in your head and I ask you to tell yourself what comfortable means. What does it feel like to be comfortable? The only stress is in your mind, and whatever you find, you let go and you can float. And now we'll move outside your head.

Focus on your jaw and your neck, with a much richer range of comforts, and you do relax and feel comfortable there. Balance or rest your head, feel relief and recognize you are thinking from these places. Feel yourself in them, and they become a part of the location of your mind.

Add the sensations of your face and relax your face. Become aware of your shoulders and let your shoulders settle. You are aware of yourself as a head and shoulders, and you can feel comfortable with this as your physical sense of self. But there is more to you and you will grow larger.

Include your torso. As you breathe, your chest expands, your sense of self grows clear with your inhale… and becomes transparent with your exhale… Your sense of location has become dynamic, it expands and contracts.

Feel your pulse. It's faint. Imagine it to make it larger. You can perceive it faintly, like a whisper or a suggestion. The sound of leaves rustling outside a window. A shadow in the periphery of your vision. Feel the pulse and the breath as the foundation of who you are. Be calm, and comfortable. Take a breath, inhale… and exhale…

Focus now on your gut, that whole area below your lungs, everything in between your front and back, from below your lungs to the cradle of your pelvis. Explore this boundary, this is a big area.

This area is full of muscles but you only sense them on the surface. You can run your mind across your skin and remember the feeling of movement there. There are muscles inside, too. And there are feelings inside, too. Let your awareness settle down, and I will count down to take you there, from five to one.

> **Five**, feeling relaxed in your mind, take this feeling expanded to your neck and shoulders.
>
> **Four**, breathing in… and out… releasing your pulse and letting your heart settle, and your blood settle, and your nerves settle.
>
> **Three**, focusing on your gut, and going into your gut, and recognizing all the awareness in your gut that does not speak to you directly.
>
> **Two**, tracing with the finger of your mind along the energy crest of digestion, just letting your attention wander peacefully into the center of your belly.
>
> **One**, settling into the center of your balance, a densely populated, microscopically aware community of careful needs and tiny voices.

Take a breath, inhale… and exhale...

You are a foreigner here but your calm presence is accepted. Like someone on a park bench surrounded by a flock of birds you move and think slowly. Your gut is quick to startle and you want it to accept you, so you must be gentle and quiet.

No matter what thoughts or feelings cross your mind, this is a matter of communication. There really are two of you: the you in your head and the you in your gut and you want them to be in communication, to share a presence, to work together.

Keep that image of yourself surrounded by a flock of birds. Amplify that sense of presence all around you. Your eyes only see one spot just as your mind only holds one thought, but your gut is a trillion thoughts and senses and you cannot share them all at once, not in the usual way. You must be calm and open and aware. Aware of the subtle and the collective. Recognize that your actions and thoughts can tip over a million balances, so you balance, sensing a cacophony in the silence, and other presences in the vacuum.

Invite your gut to come to you. Release your hold on the outside reality in order for yourself to merge with an inside reality. A separate personhood, a deeper awareness. You are a magnifying glass and your focus gets smaller, aware of smaller things, smaller sensations. Quieter noises. Tiny feelings. Minute sensations. And things get bigger around you.

Shrink to become minute, quiet, motionless, more widely aware, more sensitive hearing. Release your eyes. Release your vision. Let go of your head as your center and settle down into your gut. Release your memories of what things look like, all you remember of seeing the world through your eyes, and open to a vision from within your gut. A separate brain, a separate awareness, another world, and listen.

Your gut is a bacterial world. There are many other species, some we've heard of, like Staphylococcus, and others we haven't, like Firmicutes. They live in the lining of your intestines and there are as many bacteria in our gut as there are cells in the rest of your body. You are one consciousness and you are aware of your surroundings. They are ten trillion and each one of them is aware of their environment.

These bacteria are not human. We don't produce them and they don't share our DNA or our lifecycle. Our gut harbors a thousand different species that we know of, and hundreds of different genera of each. It is a huge and interconnected ecosystem that lives in balance and that we do little more than protect.

One species, Bacteroidetes, digests proteins and sugars. It's symbiotic in us: our lives depend on each other, and a billion Bacteroidetes live on each square centimeter of our intestines.

Lactobacillus, another large group of round-end, capsule-shaped bacteria that digest in different ways under different environments, depending on what we eat. They digest milk proteins, break down carbs, and create vitamins and acids. Left unchecked, their population can double every 20 minutes.

We hear of E. coli as creating illness and some do, but there are over a thousand strains and many are friendly, constant companions in our gut. They're all relatives, it's just that some are toxic to us. Like all relatives, some don't get along with others, and our body builds its allegiance selectively, relying on the species we support to eliminate those we don't.

Our gut harbors dozens of fungi, like Candida and Penicillium, and it's not clear if we rely on them or tolerate them. Given how well balanced the whole system is, it's likely they play a role, but we have no idea what their role is. We need and rely on all of these players.

Our immune system injects vast quantities of antibodies into the gut and the bacteria of our gut, in turn, "educates" our immune system. The T-cells and leukocytes are not born there, but that's where they develop their chemical reactance and sensitivity. Most of our immune system's activities are focused on our gut, and through this collaboration, the gut bacteria show us the world and police themselves.

A separate nervous system—the enteric nervous system, 1/10th the size of our cerebral brain—coordinates the activities of our gut producing our body's dopamine and 90% of our serotonin, neurotransmitters essential for our brain.

The gut acts as a separate endocrine system—like the hypothalamus, pituitary, and thyroid glands—to produce hormone-like chemicals that control our metabolism and regulate our moods. What's happening in our gut reflects and affects every aspect of our being, and a dysregulated gut will disrupt everything.

We'll be leaving here soon, but before we go, reach out in front of you and hold to your center, and feel that sense of center as a pillar rooted in you, something you can hold on to even when your eyes are closed. And close the eyes of your imagination, and rest any visions in your brain, and just hold on to this feeling of being centered.

Rest your mind and senses. Rest your awareness and let the details fade. Let it all fade to black as your eyes are closed and your thoughts disengaged. You are balanced and there are no feelings to disturb you. You feel as in that moment before sleep when everything is far away and you are not attached to even feeling, news, or events. Just floating in the center, quiet and calm and relaxed, feeling even and comfortable, feeling no emotion, only warmth and space.

Return back up through your body, back up into your torso where the breathing happens… feeling the movement, feeling the pulse.

Back into your spine, back into your skull where the ideas come from, but the ideas are calm now. There is only the sense of center, the sense of wonder at the expansiveness of the gut, the mystery of how things so small can be so complex, organized by nothing we're aware of, and creating a balance that has more control over us than anything we have control over.

Coming back, and counting back, moving up and into position.

One. Up into your chest and your breath. Inhale… exhale…

And **two**, to energize your spine, widen your shoulders, and stretch your neck.

Three, thinking in your head, residing in your head, feeling calm and protected.

Four, recalling the images of your two eyes, and how your mind is stereoscopic, with two visions that are almost the same.

Five, return to thinking and feeling normally. Unaware of the thoughts that bubble in your digestion, but interested in developing the intelligence you have there.

Relax and take a breath, inhale… exhale… back to mind and back to center.

---

11 – Spirit

Spiritual means purposeful: a thing's spirit is its purpose.

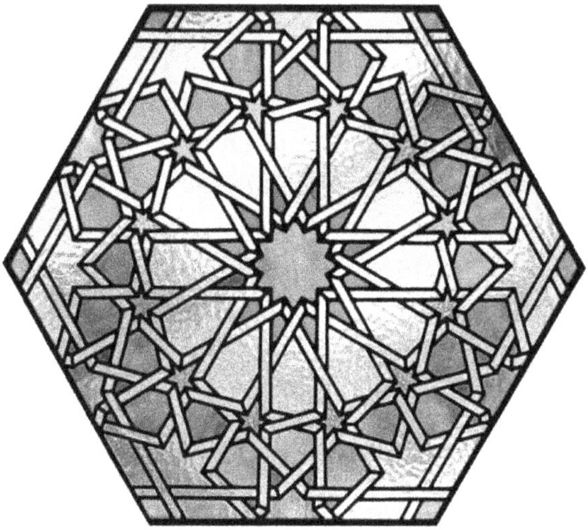

"Think of the earth as a living organism that is being attacked by billions of bacteria whose numbers double every forty years. Either the host dies, or the virus dies, or both die."
— **Gore Vidal**

The Old Science

My ideas about spirit are different enough that I don't talk about them. One half of me lives in science and the other in imagination, which I ascribe to growing up as a naturalist in a family of artists. This set me off on a trajectory shared with Friedrich Wilhelm Heinrich Alexander von Humboldt, the romantic philosopher-scientist who insisted on a combination of nature and physics, and without whom Charles Darwin would never have boarded HMS Beagle in 1831.

A response to the question of "What is the spiritual reason for the coronavirus?" appeared on David Spangler's Lorian.org blog and made me feel I was not alone. Lorian.org is seen as a spiritual organization, but it's really the White Man's indigenous tradition of herbalists and healers from before the Druids.

Scientific mysticism was evident in the spirit doctoring of Galen and Asclepius, from before metaphysics became today's religion of sales, multi-level marketing, and holy-book idols. It was evident in the 20th-century reverence for mystery held by Einstein and Schrodinger, disparaged by Richard Feynman the calculator, discarded by Steven Weinberg the mechanist, and desecrated by Ray Kurzweil the industrialist.

In "We Are The Meaning Makers," Drena Griffith (Griffith, 2020) addresses the spiritual meaning of COVID-19. She highlights the similarity between asking for meaning and asking for a reason. The meaning resides in the reason, which reflects our own meaning in the natural context. To this we might add the word "purpose," and so recognize that questioning the meaning, reason, and purpose is asking the same thing.

> "I ever desired to discern physical phenomena in their widest mutual connection, and to comprehend Nature as a whole, animated and moved by inward forces."
>
> —**Alexander von Humboldt**, *Cosmos* (Humboldt, 1846, p. xviii)

What's New?

COVID-19 is called "novel" but the human situation is more novel; more has changed in the human environment than in the virus's environment. It is the nature of people to disregard changes in their own perspective: wherever we are, always seems where we're entitled to be, and whatever we're aware of seems like all there is to be aware of.

As has been quietly declared in environmental circles, the virus's occurrence in humans is a result of our invasion into and destruction of natural habitats. The virus's transmission in humans is due to our density and mobility. If we were less dense, the transmission would be slowed within communities, and if we were less global, infection would be more localized.

Life on earth began abruptly when conditions stabilized in the seas. Soon afterward, I understand, viruses appeared. They've been with us from the start and, while we've evolved massive complexity, they haven't. But then, it's not certain that they needed to. It's three billion years from the time of the first cells and viruses now seem just as plentiful as ever, maybe more so. While our path has been a complement of increasing complexity and reproductive success, viruses have aimed for reproductive success only.

Think of life as coming in one of three forms: symbiotes, saprophytes, and parasites. The symbiotes have a mutually beneficial relationship with another life form. The saprophytes (animal saprophytes are called saprozoites) and parasites don't benefit another species. They either mine resources left behind, or extract resources from living systems.

Humans are hardly mutualistic. We farm crops and animals, but neither are natural situations. Our reliance on natural resources is saprophytic: we extract resources from non-living material. The majority of modern culture's relationship is parasitic, which is also a virus's defining relationship.

I'd like to say this virus experience will teach us something about our own parasitic relationships. Unfortunately, it's not an easy lesson, but it is some kind of lesson, nonetheless.

Maybe all parasites feel entitled to their hosts. You wouldn't feel entitled if you experienced a loss whenever you went out of balance, you'd recognize your role. It does seem that the global scale at which we're exploiting resources is at a tipping point. There is a certain balance, even for parasites.

Reflection

I'm dismayed at our culture's lack of reflection. Reflection is a prerequisite for perception and requires taking some responsibility. We're not reflective in situations where our needs are satisfied, aside from reflecting on how satisfied we feel. It takes some disruption to start people thinking. The most destructive thing about globalization is its lack of feedback. Those who benefit from and depend on the fruits of modern culture are not aware of the injuries it causes. This clearly can't go on, and it seems we're reaching the end. Might the virus be the wake-up call we need?

Questions of spirit are questions of meaning, reason, and purpose. Most scientists would agree that natural science has spirit and is spiritual in this regard. But "natural science" is not what we call science today which we associate with technology, automation, knowledge, and engineering. It's the metaphysics of Goethe or the wonder which Feynman expressed—in spite of himself—when he said, "I was born not knowing and have had only a little time to change that here and there." This kind of humility is not evident in Ray Kurzweil's attitude when he speaks as the voice of science today:

> "Our sole responsibility is to produce something smarter than we are; any problems beyond that are not ours to solve."
>
> — **Ray Kurzweil**, Director of Engineering at Google

There is a sort of natural justice, in a world out of balance, where one of the first consequences of disequilibrium is an opportunity for one of the least intelligent living things. This reflects the deep and structural nature of this disturbance. It is an imbalance created by humanity's smartest men and—all talk about gender equality aside—modern culture's progress is testosterone-fueled. If nothing else, it should show us that management cannot succeed if the environment has become dysfunctional.

> "Our imagination is struck only by what is great; but the lover of natural philosophy should reflect equally on little things."
>
> — **Alexander von Humboldt**

Spirit and Reason

I have questions that don't have answers, and they're questions about purpose and meaning and the reasons for things. I suggest our hunger for meaning and purpose is a hunger we can't satisfy, and shouldn't want to.

I've created a guided visualization called *Spirit and Reason* that explores what and how we know in order to find greater peace in the state of not knowing; to be more settled, quiet, and relieved in both the immediate present, and with regard to existential questions, also.

> "Imagination will often carry us to worlds that never were. But without it we go nowhere."
>
> — **Carl Sagan** (Sagan et al., 1980). *Cosmos*, Episode 4.

Hypnotic Session 10

Spirit and Reason audio file at: https://www.mindstrengthbalance.com/covid19-illness-illumination/

Spirit and Reason

Spirit and Reason is a hypnotic induction that requires your full attention. Do not listen to this hypnotic visualization if you are driving a car, operating machinery, or doing anything that requires your attention.

This piece explores purpose in the search for strength.

Find a relaxed position. Settle down. Close your eyes if you're ready, and if you're not, then move out and away from thoughts of the present moment and location. Raise a wall, create a distance, or sense of time that's lower, higher, closer to your center, and farther from anything that requires your engagement. Sometimes we can relax when our minds are busy pedaling forward, but we can relax more and make a different kind of progress if we stop pedaling and coast. Let gravity work for you and feel yourself coasting down into a valley of broad calm, quiet, and relief.

I have some questions that don't have answers, and they're questions about purpose and meaning and the reasons for things. We don't have deep answers for these, we have shallow answers that seem too shallow to really sail away, and too leaky to keep our feet dry. Our answers to the questions of meaning and purpose leak like old plumbing. They're the best we can do but rather insecure. It seems we can never take our eyes off them as we expect them to fail, so we baby them along, leaking doubts. Drip, drip, drip.

I suggest you take another look, and let them be. I suggest our uncertainty is a necessity, and that meaning and purpose are a hunger we can't permanently satisfy, and we shouldn't want to. They are guides not goals and we want not to settle them but recognize them as living things. It's the search for purpose and meaning that gives these to us. They are not things we find, they're things we do. Like a ride in the country, we don't do it to get anywhere.

Reason and purpose exist in their search for them, not in anything you ever find. They must always be evolving, you never catch them and you should never want to. The only purpose you'll ever find is a dead one.

Take a breath and drop down a level. Inhale… exhale… and let's spiral down below appearances into something that has more than three dimensions. We'll let the depth inside things be a fourth dimension, another realm of experience, and then we'll go on from there to higher dimensions.

Imagine you're flying, maybe in a plane or flying a plane or simply in the air, like a bird, floating on outstretched wings. In this you know some things: you know distance and volume. You know the level horizon and gravity. Leaning to the left, take a wide, descending curve and imagine what you see and feel. The horizon rises and you point down. The horizon tilts as you turn left. The landscape starts to rotate and it's somewhat disconcerting as you can't yet see what's not yet in view, and what you see in front of you keeps drifting out of view to the right.

You can't feel the turn because you're in it, so the vision of turning without the feeling of doing, makes you want to close your eyes. And you do close your eyes, and then everything feels settled again. You know you're turning. You know it but you can't see it anymore.

This is imagination so you can let things grow in imaginary directions. Imagine that the earth is opening up for you, that you are settling into the horizon and it's closing above you like a shrinking circle, like the strings of a bag. The horizon, which used to stretch around you like a great circle, is now a smaller circle up above you, getting smaller, and higher.

All around you is the vision of the surface of the earth. You can see below the surface of the earth, and at first this looks subterranean with caverns and rivers and grottos, but let it rather be the insides of things, not just below the earth's flat plain, but below the skin of everything: inside hills, mountains, forests, inside the sky, and inside of cells. All things that have things going on inside them, and are the insides of things going on around them.

There's something appealing about models of the solar system with planets making circles around each other. There is a harmony in circles, or ellipses, or whatever these orbits are. And in reality they're not circular, some don't even look like orbits as things sling-shot past to be lost in the distance never to return.

This is gravity attracting huge objects in a frictionless world, and we live on a large object and we make our own gravity, and we have no effect on the big objects, we're less than a sugar dusting. We don't participate in the gravity dance; for us the world is flat.

Breathe into a stable feeling as you sail through our field of gravity. Take a breath, inhale… exhale… and make three slow circles, settling down lower on each revolution.

One, smoothly curving to the left without effort or strain,

Two, gently rotating, simply aware of the curve of your path,

Three, inhale… and exhale… to feel larger, looser, rounder.

Recognize the earth's gravity gives us a solid place, even though the earth itself is spinning in cycles with planets, around stars, through galaxies, none of which means anything to us. Our space and our time is here, in what we experience, think, and feel. We take everything else as constant or irrelevant.

All these things make some contribution. The stars made the elements that build us, the planets soak up those elements without whose proportions we'd be poisoned. On the ancient surface of the earth, the molecules built the microbes and species that became us, that maintain us, and whose becoming we are a part of, whether we know it or not.

Think of all the parts that are in you. Our bones and muscles that we can't even imagine located or dislocated, all as one part of us, assumed and expected. And of what they're made, of cells of all kinds that don't even participate in motion or locomotion, placing, moving, orienting, or manipulating. Cells for which the universe doesn't exist, but for their own neighborhood which they cannot even imagine doing without, and what a disaster a small injury would be.

And what of inside those cells: a place for which the membrane is the edge of the known universe, which answers to the cell's brain with as many parts as there are neurons in our own, and whose function is to create a biochemistry we hardly understand beyond a few test-tube experiments and chemical elixirs. How the body supports its cells, infinitely wiser than our clueless selves.

And what of yourself, which, most of the time, seems hardly engaged with the world, twiddling its thumbs and waiting for the next meal to drift by, hardly more aware than a sponge. And that is you? What of it? Why do you even pay your mind any attention at all?

Your mind is like a fire alarm and all it does is go off. Maybe it's more like a sprinkler system since when it does go off, which happens incessantly, you spray thoughts and generally ineffectual intentions—except for eating or running toward or away from something.

And this mind you'll let disturb you? This mind you'll rely on to maintain your attitude, to keep you motivated and pointing forward? You, who barely know yourself are in charge of meaning, reason, motivation, and divine connection? With what?

This is annoying. I am annoyed. You should be annoyed, too. Our mind's judgments are Marie Antoinette reflecting on the breadless masses and saying, "Why don't they eat cake?" Hers was a head that was useless for guiding the nation. How much better is yours, beyond your skills at eating and running?

Let's relax again. Let's sink in our circles down into the macroscopic earth and the microcosmos under our noses and inside our noses. Let's be accepting of ourselves. After all, our senses are so limited and our memory so fragile. How much detail can you recall of anything? Granted, there may be many memories in your head but, like some compulsively withholding librarian, we're hardly allowed to withdraw more than one or two memories at a time.

Take three steps to accepting yourself. Take a breath. Inhale… and exhale…

> On **one**, recognize your mind as the assigned leader of your sense of self. It's not a job you volunteered for.
>
> On **two**, see all the world around you, what's immediate and what you can sometimes sense, and the infinite distances you can hardly imagine.
>
> And **three**, going inside past tissues, organs, structures, cells, membranes, organelles, microbes, viruses, molecules, functions, processes, channels, competition, alliance, mutual and parasitic, energy flowing, atoms and fields beyond any real knowing.

Don't be fooled. Don't let the experts fool you. They are foolish. We hardly know anything. You were never expected to know any of this.

Your mind is like an impotent royal family, all talk and appearance and absolutely no knowledge. Don't believe anything you think. You rely entirely on your court, and the smaller and more numerous your informants, the closer they are to what's really going on. Shame on you for guiding your life according to celebrities and ignoring the smallest people on the street. Who do you think is actually doing the work around here, the Hollywood stars or the microbes and the viruses?

Stop thinking and talking and judging and planning and start listening and feeling and asking and exploring. You're not really called upon to make pronouncements. You're not really expected to judge your self-worth. You're not even expected to be elated or depressed. You're not expected to understand love, just to explore it.

You're expected to be in balance, to be a leader, to provide the ineffable, unjustifiable, unreasonable sense of meaning and purpose on which all the parts depend. They are the material and they are interdependent. You are a ghost that can choose to be anything you want.

You don't live, you just are. You don't die, they do, our microbes, viruses, and cells, our organelles and molecules. They rely on you as we rely on the sun. You must be there for them regardless of anything. Nothing matters but your integrity to yourself, in connection, harmony, and alliance with the stars, the planets, and the galaxies.

And even this is just your imagination, built on the sense of time we share, that clocks the life cycles of our living parts and the frequencies of the nonliving. Relax the time to take in the whole orchestral maneuver.

> Count **one**, to feel a thousand microseconds, the lifetime of a molecule, and the strike of inspiration, and relax…
>
> Count to **two**, a thousand seconds, the time to reproduce genetic code and a bee finding its way home, and relax…
>
> Count to **three**, a thousand minutes, the lifetime of a white blood cell, and for you to learn something, and relax…
>
> Count to **four**, a thousand hours, the lifetime of a red blood cell, the gestation of a human, a new opportunity, and relax…
>
> Count to **five**, a thousand days, the time it takes to replace all the cells in your body and a new epoch to open in your life, and relax…
>
> Count to **six**, a thousand months, your lifetime though more than that of most and less than some, and nowhere near being important in the scheme of things, and relax…

Take a breath. Inhale… and exhale… and wrap yourself up in your memory of time and your expectations of the future in minutes, weeks, months, and years. It's all distorted through a lens that makes the immediate seem all-important.

Our impressions of almost everything are logarithmic: distance, brightness, sensation, intention, time, you name it. Everything seems huge and important in the present, at the moment, and on the surface and then gradually fades away into the numbing distance which we grumble about like a parliament of democrats and republicans.

> **Five**… **four**… **three**… **two**… **one**.

And what of spirit, meaning, and reason? Must we have an answer? What makes you think we can find these things? What makes you think we'd know them if we saw them? And of all the things that might or could be, how are we to judge?

It's all in how you feel, and how are you going to feel? Whose agenda will you follow: your parents', your country's, your ancestors', or something of your own? I can assure you, you are the best shepherd of your own best interests. Even if you do it badly and without thinking, it's not thinking that you rely on. It doesn't take thinking to have memories, and it doesn't take much thinking to respond to them. How you respond is built into you. It resides in your structure and guides the expression of your genetics.

You have that potential. But recognize you didn't start with your first memories and you won't be ending with your last. Your flock is bigger than you, and your obligation is far wider than what you can eat and where you can run to. You don't need an education, authorization, religion, or family. You already have those things. What you do with your mind is window dressing. Don't confuse the icing on the cake for the bread of sustenance. Let your feelings guide you.

Take a breath. Inhale… exhale…

You've pushed your boundaries inward, outward, and time-ward. You've added three dimensions and you can keep them. We think of dimensions as things we measure with a ruler and around which we can rotate and redirect, like the turning of the earth or our sweep around the horizon.

Dimensions have other aspects and you want to keep them. We mostly live in two dimensions, living on a flat surface and inferring depth from a flat image of the world. We expand ourselves to three, through our imagination of flight and our ability to view remotely.

Expand yourself into the realm of larger sizes, of boundaries like the weather and the ocean, volumes and expansive surfaces. Enter the microscopic through the tendrils of your connection to the processes of cells and membranes, to the urges of the biochemical, microbic, and viral.

Dilate yourself in time to follow the quick and the slow. Recognize that in each domain, along each dimension, there are different reasons and meanings, some long-lasting and others over in an instant.

These things change. They are a currency and you trade them, trading one good meaning for another. Like the change in your pocket, there are large bills and small coins and you are a piggy bank of their collection. You don't need meaning; you are meaning. You are the reason, you have the spirit. No one can give it to you. You don't need to ask permission, charity, or absolution.

Bring these meanings and reasons back. They are your ancestry and extension into the future. Whenever you tilt your head your ears tell you of the shift in your horizon, a measure of your space and relationship. Whenever you tilt your head your relationship turns and you feel the force of gravity and its reason. Meaning lies in motion and direction and relationship. You have these things, and they arise when needed. Wait for them.

Tilt now to the right and make three circles back around. Three large wide circles. Three large gentle circles. Leaning to the right, watch the horizon begin to cycle around you, like the hands on a clock, and you can speed them up. Inhale, rotating; 15-seconds, 30-seconds, exhale, 45-seconds, and back around to 12.

Around another circle, inhale, rotating: 15-seconds, 30-seconds, exhale, 45-seconds, and back around to 12.

And then the last rotation, straightening up, leveling the horizon, slowly rotating like a playground carousel. Inhale… 15-seconds, 30-seconds, slowing down, coasting to a gentle turn. 45-seconds, hardly moving, moving just enough to make it 'round, and coming back to stop just at 12. And you're back and you're still, and you're larger, and deeper, and of greater duration.

The search for reason and meaning is the reason and meaning we search for. We're built to search and not to know or find. We're built to expand and find purpose in simply looking, regardless of what we find or think we find. Regardless of what we're worth or think we're worth. Support yourself, everything depends on it. Be gentle and aware, present and alert.

Open your eyes. Open your ears. Open your heart. Hear what speaks to you in the wind, in the rotation of the world outside and in the microcosmos, and remember.

12 – Ecology Big and Small

Ecologies balance and change. Every part contributes

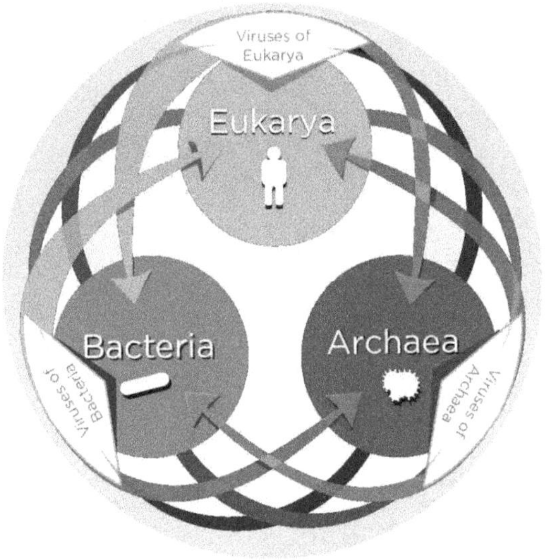

"We are like butterflies who flutter for a day and think it is forever."
— **Carl Sagan**

Identity

We think we know all of what we are, and control all of what we do. We say we're responsible and entitled to our authority, and so we're due life, liberty, and the pursuit of happiness, and not just from our government but from nature. An infection seems unfair, even unjust. But nature doesn't agree, and we can't win the argument, so we view the virus as separate and evil.

We have little authority at the microscopic level of the virus, aside from taking care of ourselves. But then, with regard to our environment, we don't act responsibly, either. We think of ourselves as individuals, but we are an ecosystem inside and out. We are larger in our impact, smaller in our importance, older than our immediate ideas, and less in control of our situation and our fate than we believe.

It's not clear whether our sense of identity is even necessary for our survival. Most animals, to which we grant little self-identity or rights of life, not only survive but harmoniously prosper. It would be irrelevant to argue that humans achieve greater life, liberty, or happiness than other animals. We take it for granted.

Ecology

For one hundred years after Alexander von Humboldt introduced the idea of ecology, it was just an idea, a theory, a fantasy. In the 1970s, we started to see some consequences in urban pollution, limited resources, and effects of a global nature. Ecology, which has been a political football match since the time of Malthus, became a populist slogan with back-to-the-earth movements represented by The Whole Earth Catalog, Greenpeace, Earth First! and others.

These movements were a hodgepodge of science, cultural change, anti-corporatism, communalism, and romanticism. They lacked a sustaining plan, goal, community, or economy and, because of this, they lacked unity. Ecology of this sort said, "Save our resources!" with the unspoken addendum of "… for us." This is not ecology; it's sustainable planning engaging in a group hug in which no one is serious. No one knew what was going on in the 70s.

To this day, there is no comprehensive definition of ecology. Small "e" ecology amounts to doing bad things less: conservation. Big "e" Ecology has tried to define itself as Deep Ecology, a kind of global vision, but this falls short. It falls short because it still has no plan or goal. Ecology is not separable from the whole ecosystem, which includes the wills of people and the wiles of governments.

Real ecology is a way of being, not a way of thinking, because being involves the feedback to maintain itself. Because of its immediacy, being connects with balance and is aware of it. All real ecologies involve feedback between the whole of their interacting parts. Complex, feedback systems are nonlinear and behave unpredictably.

Thinking, or strategizing, is linear because it involves prediction and assessment, and we can do that with linear models. Stratagems are not dynamic, they are revised, and they are incremental. Strategies do not have the kind of built-in evolutionary mechanisms found in ecologies. You cannot commit to a strategy for navigating a nonlinear system, and our social and political systems do not work well, or do not work at all, where there is no strategy. How can you sell a long-term plan for something you cannot predict?

Until we, as a species, have an awareness of all the parts that we affect, we can't plan a sustainable ecology. Until we have flexible social and political structures that remain intact under radically changing conditions we won't be able to maintain stability over the course of dramatic change.

Virions

To the virus, we are not people, we're just an oasis of resources in a barren landscape. For them, or it, we are everything and, were they religious, they might revere us as the gods on which they depend.

> "It was an exciting moment… People realized we didn't know anything about microbial biodiversity."
>
> — **Jean-Michel Claverie**, evolutionary microbiologist, 2003 co-discoverer of Mimivirus.

What does it feel like to be the prey instead of the predator? Are we any less important because our survival is not assured? If the survivor is recognized as the superior form, what of the virus which will never die?

We shepherd our external ecosystem and our internal biota. The viruses are the wolves. If we understood the necessary role the virus played, could we collaborate? Do the caribou feel sympathy for the wolves?

The wolves keep the herd strong in several ways. First, they remove the weak so the strong prevail, improving the herd. Second, their threat compels collaboration, communication, and consensus. And third, when the ecosystem is balanced, resources are used effectively.

We're in a similar position. The virus does endanger the weak. We might object that one's immunity doesn't reflect one's importance but, in the end, the virus is the arbiter of fitness. If we valued our elders more, we wouldn't warehouse them in vulnerable nursing homes. That's society's choice. Are we going to do anything differently now?

What of our strength? We can improve the emotional and nutritional quality of our lives. The virus is a test of our health decisions, many of which we've been lamenting and ignoring for years. Many of our decisions have served short-term desires over long-term interests.

Unlike wolves to caribou, the virus gives us things. In fact, viruses have contributed greatly to our evolution. Viruses are the only organism that shares its genetic code to both create mutualistic relations and to transport genetic material between organisms. Viruses share genes across the entire tree of life. Many of our genes have been acquired from viruses. Our mammalian placenta has a viral origin. Eight percent of human DNA is of viral origin.

> "We use DNA from viruses to do things that are essential to our own survival, scientists are finding. Somehow, we have managed to domesticate some of these invaders."
>
> — **Carl Zimmer**, the *New York Times*

When attacked, we circle the wagons. Is the virus's ability to penetrate our defenses a reflection of its strength or our weakness? Surviving illness involves more than running under the skirts of medicine or government. How healthy is it that the most we know about our bodies is what we see on TV news?

The virus is not a personal or social assault—it's an environmental event. More than an event, it is a consequence of our choices. If we don't see it as an aspect of something for which we're responsible, then we will not only fail to control our future but we will also fail to create a sustainable environment.

> "It's not an either-or—are these things good or bad? It's a lot more complicated than that... We're barely at the beginning of this research."
>
> — **Dr. Aris Katzourakis**, virologist

Humboldt

Alexander von Humboldt, living in the first half of the 19th century, was more celebrated in his lifetime than any scientist in history; more widely followed than Newton or Einstein and on a par with how we now view Leonard da Vinci. And although both da Vinci and Humboldt are considered the greatest of scientists, they did not practice what we call science today. Both of these great "scientists" lived in a time before the term "scientist" existed, as the word was coined in 1834. We worship science now, but we ignore what it really means.

As the model for Indiana Jones, Humboldt did more than anyone to make science a household word. An effusive romantic, Humboldt bridged heart and mind by presenting science as life. His effort was to bring intellect and emotion together, a project that long preceded him in the conflicting works of Newton, Bacon, Goethe, and others.

> "For Humboldt... 'objectivity' meant embracing mind and imagination—intellect, poetry, and emotion—as multiple modes of access that allow humans to participate in the grand unfolding of the cosmos."
>
> — **Laura Dassow Walls, Stephen T. Jackson, & Mark W. Person,** from *Views of Nature, Alexander von Humboldt* (Walls et al., 2014)

It's fair to say that Humboldt's discoveries, and the ideas he endorsed, were too much for the world. This was before Darwin's theory of evolution—which Humboldt directly inspired—in a world dominated by colonialism. Humboldt claimed all peoples were equal, and all things were related with connections at every scale. He was not limiting himself to a small or local sense, but incorporating all humans, plants, animals, geography, meteorology, and astronomy. The implications that the whole world is a balanced ecosystem went unheeded, until today.

It was Humboldt's five-volume *Cosmos* that led Carl Sagan—150 years later, in his own production of *Cosmos*—to declare, "The nitrogen in our DNA, the calcium in our teeth, the iron in our blood, the carbon in our apple pies were made in the interiors of collapsing stars. We are made of star-stuff."

The Next Step

Recognizing star-stuff is not enough. The rocks are made of star-stuff, but they don't have the responsibility that we do. Even our complex structure does not explain us. It's our relationships to things that define us.

Rise above the idea that things can be understood in terms of their components. The solar system is made of dust, and it has created a sun, planets, and an environment that fosters life. Same stuff, different result. After you die, you are made of the same stuff as when you were alive. There's no "thing" missing, but you are missing because all of your relationships are gone: you are in the relationships of things.

For as long as people have been thinking, we've been breaking things down. Even after our most fundamental science tells us there's nothing at the smallest levels, we keep looking. Rearranging the equation $E=mc^2$ gives you the equation mass equals energy divided by the speed of light squared: it's all energy and light. What seems like matter is actually the energy of relationships!

Relationships have effects that extend beyond the systems that are related. Such relationships between things don't end at the boundaries of the things. A virion is small, but the virus is as large as the ecosystem perhaps bigger than our own ecosystem, since the virus can cross between species. The virus is as big as the relationships it creates.

The entirety of the virus is one entity. The virions are all clones who depend on their relationship to our cells. As long as we are blind to their existence as part of the ecology we have created, they will continue to mine us as a resource. We are a resource they have no reason to conserve.

You can change your relationship to your cells, how you define yourself, and how you relate to your environment. By finding a deeper connection at all levels, you reshape the structure of the relationships and the matter created from them. It isn't one domain or the other. This isn't just a microscopic, personal, or social issue; the ecology is all of them in relationship with each other.

You will not defeat the virus. You will not conquer your emotions. You will not subjugate the environment. The virus, your emotions, and the environment all require a balance, an alliance, and you learn this alliance by creating it.

All doing starts with a vision, an image: it is what can be imagined. All insight and direction come from there. You must create the ecosystem in your imagination, like a hologram, as something you can recall, recreate, and re-experience.

I have created a guided visualization called *Ecology*, which guides you toward experiencing yourself as a system in a larger system, and to think beyond mechanism to synergy and balance. To act in harmony with our environment, we must feel our environment and act in consonance with our feelings. *Ecology* is not just acting to maintain the balance; it's maintained by understanding at a deeper level that it is the right thing.

Hypnotic Session 11

Ecology audio file at: https://www.mindstrengthbalance.com/covid19-illness-illumination/

Ecology

Ecology is a hypnotic induction that requires your full attention. Do not listen to this hypnotic visualization if you are driving a car, operating machinery, or doing anything that requires your attention.

Ecology is about finding a larger, older, and stronger frame of mind.

In this piece, I'd like you to consider ecology not as a thought, idea, or theory but as a way of being, or as a sense of being. If you're of European descent, or you've internalized the European attitude that dominates, then you'll think of ecology in much the same way as we talk about nature, as a kind of optional idea that's both out of reach and in need of revision. No one wants nature in their lives full blown because no one lives entirely in nature anymore.

Well, some might, but most of us—living on the grid, in cities, with jobs and professions, regulated by states and provinces with rules and representatives—don't. Few of us clock by the sun, navigate by the stars, survive by the weather, and endure nature's tantrums. Those solitary woodsmen, farmers, fishermen, ranchers, trappers, and miners are vanishing and are rarely seen outside of story, myth, or family albums. Nature is becoming a fairy tale, and we treat ecology as one, too. Our current direction to read, study, analyze, and research will not change that. It will only make it more so. We come back to it only through experience.

There are subtle things that happen when you move away from nature firsthand, and reduce your role to that of an outsider. When you lose a personal relationship with your environment—a relationship with spirit and ceremony—you lose a language and a means to communicate with others.

You lose a means to understand and a means to control yourself in your larger and less well-known environment; you become isolated, with less feeling and intuition.

When the balance is upset or when you are upset—as there may never have really been a balance—you're left feeling like a victim. This piece is about regaining a human role for yourself. Finding a place for spirit and ceremony.

Find a relaxed position, somewhere you can settle in and forget about things without being disturbed. It could be a chair or a bed, alone in your house or, just as good, it could be on a bus, train, or subway where you're assured no contact or connection. Make sure you have 30 minutes before you need to get up.

This doesn't require anything special except that your environment does not intrude, and does not demand your attention, and it will not bother you. Like when you're really tired, when you make up your mind you need to sleep, you can fall asleep anywhere, under any condition.

Relax, now, those places in your body where you hold stress. Physical stress is mental ideas that have been over tightened. Conflicts you've placed in your body because you can't keep them all in your mind at once, but your body can hold them—as many as you want—and you don't worry about forgetting them.

Touch in your thoughts each of those areas that feels grey or black, that are hard or lack sensation, or feel tired, dull, or achy. Make an inventory of those places where you so often feel stress that you tend not to feel them at all. These are places you would stretch and air out, or permanently remove, but you don't get around to it. Maybe it's the base of your neck, or a band around your scalp, or your waist, or your feet. Maybe it's that feeling in your throat of needing to say something but not knowing what to say. That need to shout without knowing what to shout about.

Settle into a quiet place of mind. Imagine you're descending into your body as if you were going down into a subterranean cavern. Not a dark or narrow cave, but a huge, honeycombed space lit by glowing orbs and crystals. Just create this vision as if it were a movie, starting as you settle into deeper feelings. Measure your way down by counting.

Imagine you're at the surface on a clear day and the entrance is a dark, tall, but narrow opening in the earth.

> At the count of **ten** you step down the first step, feeling your breath, moving down.
>
> **Nine**, you move through the opening, still descending on cool, worn stones.
>
> **Eight**, it's gotten dark now as the light is dim and your eyes aren't used to it.
>
> **Seven**, move mostly by feel, sound, and balance, a combination of echos and the ringing in your ears.
>
> **Six**, take a breath and relax as your eyes become accustomed and you see spaces taking form.
>
> **Five**, see the faint points of light, shaded colors in the distance, and some points next to you.
>
> **Four**, move into the cavern where you can hear the space, the depth before, above, and around you.
>
> **Three**, the ground has become flat and you can better see the faint light of glowing crystals.
>
> **Two**, slower movement lets the sounds and spaces resonate, solid but reflecting, detailed, curious, and inviting.
>
> **One**, feeling something deeper opening, a felt sense of connection and knowing. The feeling sweeps past you like a breeze.

Move through your body and take an inventory of places of special feelings. These places are numerous. Some might stand out and, in fact, some might pain you and others make you happy. Others might be occasional, good ones that make you jump or hunger, and bad ones like heartburn, or sore feet. Some might slow you down and others give you pleasure, confidence, or strength. Locate the sensations around those feelings, the tissues, joints, muscles, and organs in these neighborhoods. Make connections between these places in your mind. This is a map of your territory, one you wander around throughout the day, like a game of snakes and ladders.

If you're old, you might think these things are wearing out. If you're young, you might think these things need more exercise. If you believe what people tell you, you might think these are just what you get, unchangeable things like eyesight, emotions, or intelligence. It's not true: all these things are changeable by force of will alone. Just let go of the things to which you're attached.

Feel yourself floating in the cavern, through the space, moving past lights and sounds. The space is getting larger and falling below you. You're rising above the walls, rising out of a twisting canyon, with muffled surfaces below and an echoless sky above. Rising out of the canyon into a wide and darkened high-mountain desert, a moonless night-scape dotted with the dark shapes of trees and outcrops, and the gentle sound of a warm, dry wind.

Recognize, again, in your body the places you store feelings: the good ones, the bad ones, the joyful and the troubling, and place these feelings into the wide landscape that's around you, as if the landscape was your body, as both your body and the landscape merge in your imagination.

Place your shoulders in the image of two, connected peaks against the horizon. Place your back in the crust of the earth through which the canyon passes. And the other places, your stomach and your organs all find a match in the landscape as trees or forests, plains, or oases. And your breath is the wind, and there are animals, though you can't see them. And everything is alive or has life on it. Bacteria, insects, birds and mammals, and microbes like viruses, floating or attached, growing or waiting.

You are filled with living things. Do you realize that each of your cells is a separate thing, with a separate awareness, process, role, and lifespan? Each organ a collaboration of millions of cells, operates, regulates, and collaborates with millions of foreign microbes as well as native cells, tissues, and organs. And isn't it amazing that you aren't aware of them as anything? You can't hear them talking, negotiating, organizing or responding. So imagine you can, and then maybe you will.

Take a breath and rise up farther, higher into the sky, so that you can see the curve of the earth and other landscapes in the farther distance. Rising through the dry haze of the nighttime the air becomes clear and cold, and you can feel the waves in the wind and the scent of the air.

To the left, a great flat area might be an ocean. To the right, a mottled deeper black might be a forest. Flashes on the dark horizon are lightning spilling from dark clouds. No sound, just flashing summer lightning, illuminating a cloud-bank and then fading again.

The desert is a valley and there are ridges around it, and the moon is coming up. A silver shine is building in the eastern sky. The moon will be rising. It's a cold, blue silver disk, a blinding white against an empty darkness.

Imagine the wind is your breathing, and the flashes are your pulse. Your feelings are the textures of the landscape grading into each other, separate but all in relationship. Take a deep breath as the wind blows through you and the lightning flashes in the distance. And exhale as the warm wind calms into the pulsing silence.

Inhale… exhale… Relax and lose your shape as your pieces float away into the landscape. You are the forest and the hills, plains and plateau. Your blood courses through the landscape, and your liquids are the aquifers below the surface. Darkness is your awareness of yourself, entirely intact and fully informed without sunlight or vision to guide you.

The moon is rising, and you are rising, and a blinding white light punctures the horizon, too bright to look into, but too soft to caste but faint shadows. And you turn your attention away from it, turning your back to it, and you flee toward the dark forest and lightning clouds in the west, rising higher and faster, faster than the earth turns, and the moon sinks again as you free yourself from your earthly body, faster than a sunray, faster than the northern lights.

Relax into the sky, a broad and welcoming home, just the right size to breathe freely, softly. Inhale long and slow, letting your vision settle inward to emotion, and exhale a stardust of ancient images and celestial places. Going deeper, three… two… one… to a place you rarely visit except in your dreams and no one else would understand.

There are buildings around you in this starlit void. Clouds or banks or islands with buildings, places that feel familiar and places you can't recall. And they might seem classical with columns or modern with wide windows, courtyards, piazzas, promenades, gardens, ornate, simple, wild, oriental, cultivated, overgrown, or organic.

Relax and take it in, the calm yet unfamiliar, the strange yet idyllic, neither young nor old, recent nor distant, timeless, like your deeper sense of self. A mind-scape of intention. A place built of other things and places, like a higher dimension. Like flying above your body's landscape, an overview and disconnection. Here is another place of higher relationships between species and lifetimes, habitats and evolution.

Approach one of these buildings, find an interesting one. Wrap yourself in a body so that you can touch the floor and pass through the door. And make this a comfortable body though it may be unfamiliar, of a different shape or weight or color or sex, clothed in robes or wraps, jacketed or even naked, perhaps formless. Pass through the doorway into a library of history and possibilities. The entry is large with desks and tables and corridors, rows, and stacks leading in all directions, maybe shelves of books, or banks of data, monitors, readers, viewers, indexed and arranged by place and history or future species, real, possible, virtual outcomes of different lineage, location, and scale.

There are guides like librarians, maybe people, entities, echos, virtual, or embedded in the medium. Someone seems to be guiding you, putting ideas into your head, explanations that seem to arise wordlessly showing you how to navigate through the texts, the halls of data, the chaos of interconnections.

This library keeps changing, rearranging and re-indexing, nothing seems to move but nothing looks the same twice. It's bigger than you can grasp and organized in a fluid and dynamic way with things grouped by size and shape, keyed by words, sounds, color, movement, and feeling. Your mind is small and linear, holding one thought at a time and then moving to another, but here everything is connected through time, space, structure, progress, regress, series and sequence. It's a picture of the real world laid out with all its possibilities, everything hidden exposed, all connections followed to all their consequences.

You're presented with one small book that has your name on it. You hold it in your hands. It is so small, so ordinary. Bound in a faded green cover, it looks old but it is firm and intact. You open it, but it is not what you expect. It opens like a pop-up book, unfolding in three dimensions with leaves in all directions, postage-stamp-sized pictures at all angles. These pictures are moving holograms, each footnoted with links like threads into the surrounding space, winding in and through and beyond it, some thin or thick, faint like spider threads or shimmering like heat haze into other dimensions, connecting to other books and people, times, places, events and outcomes.

The book has dimensions of colors and sounds. Electric fields with waves of possibilities and scatter plots of combinations. Pictures of different futures and different pasts, possible, contingent, and historic. There are pictures of your youth that you remember, and pictures of other youths that you don't. People you recognize and many you can't.

Follow these forward to the present and you see references to the virus. Thread lines and fields like waves lead out in more biological and microscopic directions, toward images and languages you cannot understand, and places that are internal or microscopic and beyond your ability to navigate or comprehend.

For these confounding paths, the guide speaks directions into your mind, directing you to run your attention along lines and planes, like surfing with your mind, to see different relationships create and disappear along with different consequences that arise or fade away.

You have the choice of following one or the other, though you don't know if you're reviewing a real past, a possible past, or a possible future, or maybe the real future. Each has a different feeling, not just a different story. It's as if you play a different role, becoming a different person depending on the relationships you choose. And you understand you can be different, and it's another thing to be outside of the familiar, and there are points of view that make sense only if you engage them. You cannot see all possibilities from any one perspective.

Relax and sink into the buzzing, endless complexity. Don't try to watch or resolve, just run your eyes over it, like a spotlight over a city, or a telescope over the heavens. As in a dream, emotions come and go, appearing reasonable in the moment but making no sense a moment later.

Take a breath and relax the urge to remember or recollect the details. You'll remember the feelings inside you, and those feelings will be your guidance. You don't need to know the details, your body will know how to achieve the paths you feel drawn to.

Some paths you can follow and seem to understand, others are too strange and foreign, or are uncomfortable, or incomprehensible. Yet even these might be available to you if you accepted the formless chaos they seem to present. Perhaps you could navigate even the microscopic worlds.

Step back and see that there are larger worlds, too. Larger than the book you're holding, of which the book is just a page, and which appear in many places in these larger books, echoing and repeating like fractals, blinding like the rising moon in a house of mirrors. These larger books are harder to see because they have no single form but always many. They are larger ecosystems of larger relationships, not just between agents at one time, but over different spans of time, achieving more than one purpose.

Take a breath, relax. You can let go of the books, they won't fall, they are embedded in the space so that you move them by just shifting your body. And you relax and let go of your need to know, and things settle into rhythms of their own, more than you can control. And the less you try, the more you see and the better you feel. The more information comes past you, the more you understand the whole of it, in spite of the multiplicity of its details.

This is a lesson. You are a student. Life is your homework. There is no one answer. These books are the relationships. Your book is a catalog of your possibilities. Your task is to explore many and find the best for you, in relation to how you see the links and the power you feel in these links and the larger, longer, deeper possibilities they uncover.

Maybe you'll fall ill, now or later, maybe you won't. A hundred different paths, a million different outcomes. You have a choice now, and you'll have a role later. Don't believe the story you're told, the books have no one storyline. Don't demand certainty or sequence because some outcomes don't provide these in the moment. Don't let your story be captured in a story that is not yours, or is not meaningful to you. No matter what any story offers, follow those paths that are yours, always meaningful, present, and having purpose.

One page comes out in your hand, the page of the present, a page of holograms or a hologram itself. It shows different pictures from different angles and it connects, like a jigsaw puzzle piece, to other puzzles at all sides. You can take this page with you, to remind you that who you are is just one facet of a larger set of facets of units. And this page melds into the palm of your hand, like the lines on your palm, like a tattoo.

Relax into purpose. Every purposeful effort, done with care, flowers in one way or another. Seeds are always formed which you may or may not see planted or germinating. Some purposes create a million seeds, like a weed or a virus, but you, too, can follow paths that spawn a million seeds.

Look for your wisdom and ways to broadcast it. These ways may not be obvious and they may not be what's advertised. Look for the small things, the obvious things, the easy things. Those are things you can do a lot of and that will affect many. Don't act for yourself because there is no "yourself." Yourself alone is yourself without meaning or mass. You are beyond that, you don't need that.

The guide collects the books from you. The book with your name on it returns not to a shelf, but to a cloud of other names, a small planetary system, orbiting around larger books with the names of locations, futures, families, and relationships. Children, relatives, histories, memories and recollections.

You find yourself floating above the building, above the gardens. Floating into another perspective, back into the moonlight-filled space, back into the stars.

Let yourself settle and let movement take you, to drift with the course of events back toward the landscape, the textured desert, the starlit sky and its stormy horizon.

Below you are the highland desert, the sandstone canyon, the shadows of stunted pitch pines and acacia trees. Settle down into the cradle of the canyon, and the sinuous curves of its waterworn walls, deeper into the crystal cavern of silent echoes, pulsing lights and glowing gems.

Touch down on the cavern floor and begin to walk, again. The slope rises gently and broad stairs form. The steps rise as you approach the narrow entrance, and you reach out to touch the walls, and you see the page of the book still shimmering on the palm of your hand. You can touch the walls, the page of your book is inside you, inside your glass palm, connected to your inner system, a window outward and inward onto the possible.

Climbing up the steps you come out into the desert before dawn. The wind has stopped as the Earth turns between night and day, paused between its exhale and inhale. Pink dawn rising in the east, mixing overhead toward purple darkness in the west.

You walk along a well-worn path now, with the sky turning from deep blue to azure. And your glass hand is normal again, except when you look directly into your palm, and you can see the hologram of possibilities.

Come back to the present, connect to the whole through a small window, feel calm and comfortable. Ready for your next stop or next step.

Five, **four**, **three**, **two**, **one**, and you're back where you were, in your bed, on a chair, in a bus, train, or subway. You're present but softer, wider, and without any of your usual hard edges. Those have been worn away, like the dog ears of a well-read book, a page of which you can see whenever you look into the palm of your hand.

Close your hand. Feel the joints and palm and wrist. Take a breath. Inhale through your palm and exhale from all your pores being comfortable, centered, and present.

---

13 – Consilience: Reason and Emotion

A lesson in the reconciliation of opposites and the shepherding of resources.

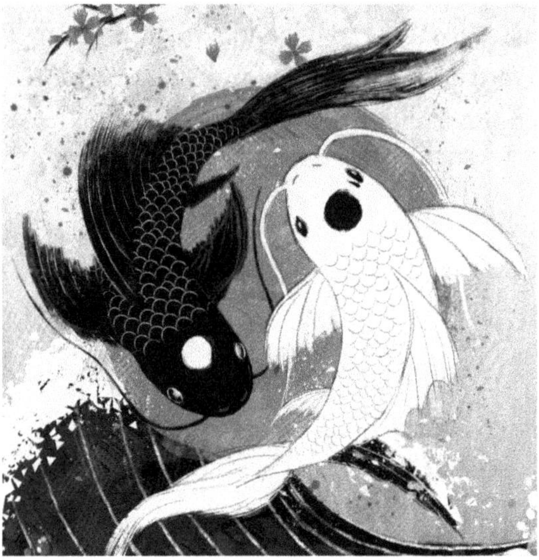

"Salvation is not a reward for the righteous, its is a gift for the guilty."
— **Steve Lawson**, author

Learning

Learning is change. We use the term "learning" to mean something conscious or intentional, but even if we're unmotivated or the change is unintentional, learning still changes us. We also talk about machine learning, and we can think of species learning, or environmental learning.

When we think about learning, we think about teaching, as the two seem complementary. But who teaches a machine, species, or environment? In truth, while learning describes something that happens, teaching is a concept we've invented. What we call teaching is an act of changing the environment so that learning, which happens anyway, happens differently.

Teaching is interference for the purpose of bringing things to the learner's attention. There has long been a confused discussion as to whether better learning requires better teachers or better learners. We observe that better performance, happiness, security, and control follow from better learning, and we presume it comes from better teaching.

We focus on the credentials of teachers but not the quality of teaching if, indeed, teaching really exists as a quality. Certainly, some situations are more conducive to learning than others. Some of those more conducive situations involve people designated as teachers, but, as most people would agree, the most important learning doesn't involve people who see their role as teachers.

For example, a college student learns many things, but most of what he or she learns doesn't happen in classes taught by teachers. Similarly, most of what parents and warriors learn is not learned in school but on the battlefront of childrearing and conflagration. What we learn is embedded in our character. Who teaches this?

Evolution is a learning process. Evolution can be described in many ways, and natural selection—the old Darwinian idea—is the generally accepted description. Natural selection does not arise from basic physical laws, so I don't believe it, but it's easy to understand and simulate in a lab or machine.

Natural selection is anthropomorphic. It's what we do when we think logically: we recognize choices, test the choices, accept some and reject others. Few things in the natural world operate in this fashion. Logical natural selection does not describe evolution in real systems, and this is quite important. If evolution—or learning—did follow logic, exceptions would never occur. For this reason, random mutations must be added for natural selection to work.

Ecological systems learn through nonlogical means. We might call them statistical, many-threaded, or holographic. Most learning in nature occurs in a chaotic fashion in which old structures collapse and new ones emerge. Much of our own learning is done by nonlogical means. There's more to our learning process than what's rational, because there is so much more to us than our rational awareness.

I suggest using the word rational instead of logical because we almost never use logic. Logic rests on certainty while reason requires only the plausible, and that's usually all we have. We develop strategies and program learning machines based on what's plausible.

This happens at a superficial level. Making strategies is how we test things, but it's not how we learn things. Most of our learning is done by association, metaphor, and emotion. There are good reasons for this, as it allows for creativity.

COVID-19 is a learning situation. The chaos the virus has fomented—disorganized as it might be—is a learning environment. The "solution" to the COVID-19 "problem" is not a rational strategy, because none of the rational strategies available are big enough. COVID-19 is here because we've been thinking too small for too long.

What the virus is exposing is the reality of our social and environmental structure, not the reasoned personal and national identities we believe define us. And how have we been deceived into learning a flawed version of our place in the world's ecology? We designated our parents, and designed our teachers and leaders to teach this to us.

Reason

I offer you three related points of view: physics, neuroscience, and behavior. As you move from the first to the second to the third, the rules governing behavior degenerate toward chaos.

Part of this is historical. It's certainly easier to learn, teach, and navigate systems that are well-ordered. It's easier to write history according to the fiction that the causes and events made some kind of sense, and one version of events provided the rationale for the narrative. But as one's awareness broadens, the reality that chaos is a dominant force becomes more evident.

When you study any historical event, you "go down the rabbit hole." This means that what's going on under the surface is unlike what we see on the surface. It also refers to the nature of rabbit holes as full of passageways, rooms, twists, turns, and alternative destinations. The rabbit-hole metaphor is a more accurate description of history and, consequently, a better model for learning.

Things are organized and logical in isolation. The number of choices can be limited. As systems get larger and more components interact, we're quickly overwhelmed by choices, forces, and outcomes. Chaos is just a label for a situation we no longer understand.

We can't understand big, complicated systems because we cannot contain them in our awareness. The human brain may be the most complicated system in the universe, but it can barely cope with the reality it confronts. You can barely remember a string of more than seven digits, and you can hold only one thought in your head at one time. We're underpowered, given the problems we face.

We're starting to understand that our minds can operate holistically and that most of our learning happens this way. This is what dreams are, and this is what we spend all of our sleeping time doing, though we remember next to none of it. We are probably also dreaming while we are awake, without being aware of it. We actually have many mental processes going on at once, with the conscious, logical process being just the tip of the iceberg.

Understanding our experience of COVID-19—our understanding of anything, really—depends on our incorporating multiple perspectives. No one perspective is complete, and no one story is complete.

Looking for a "complete description" is a dead end. There is none because the virus lies at the intersection of many systems. Many of these systems were not designed, or did not evolve, to respond to this infection. The virus has disrupted medicine, politics, economics, science, genetics, and ecology, not to mention physiology and metabolism. No story written from any of these points of view will be complete.

Awareness

We think of attention as an action, as "to pay attention," but it's also a state, as "to be attentive." We identify attention with awareness and apply the binary quality of awareness—of either being aware or unaware—with a binary quality of attention—either paying attention or not.

> "My experience is what I agree to attend to."
>
> — **William James**, PhD, psychologist

Watching brain states reveals that attention lies on a spectrum. One can only pay attention to what one can discern, and discernment requires change. Our minds need change in order to maintain focus, which is why we use rosaries, mantras, dialog, legends, and celebrations to hold our attention. It's next to impossible to meditate on nothing; you can do it only by going into an intermittent state of thoughtless awareness, a kind of listening state with distant boundaries.

As your brainwaves speed up you become more attuned to rapid changes and, I believe, memories of shorter duration. Slower brainwaves enable you to be more aware of slower changes and, I suspect, memories of longer duration.

The character of your brainwaves changes with your situation, your energy level, and the time of day. You can also train your brainwaves. With practice, you can voluntarily control what you're aware of. This hyper-focus supports higher-level performance (Thomas, 2018).

The character of your thought and speech follows the nature of your focus. The range of your brainwaves—which is to say, your focus—defines your personality, your responses to your environment, the ideas you hold, and the friends you make.

To one extent this is obvious: when your brainwaves stop, you die. But to another extent it's profound: you can change your awareness. We don't know how much control you can gain, or the full range of characteristics controlled by it; but controlling your brainwaves controls your ability to attend. You can voluntarily become more aware, engaged, and insightful.

Identity

You are what you're aware of. This is quite a different thing from your personality.

Your personality determines your success in your interactions with other people, but not your control over your environment. Patience, temperateness, and good humor will help you solve problems, but intelligence, insight, and artistry exist in a different realm.

Our personality is shaped by school, work, and society, and is a measure of our maturity. With our personality, we navigate social situations. The major focus of modern schooling—which is to say nonsectarian schooling of the last 200 years—is on the shaping of personality.

Our awareness—which includes intelligence, insight, and artistry—is not considered to be a learned skill. Yet our awareness determines to a large degree our ability to navigate our environment. My experience training people's brains, and the whole field of neurofeedback therapy, is all about enabling people to become more aware.

You learn through feedback. You stretch your awareness by encountering elements outside your full awareness but partially within reach. You typically have, or can be directed to have, a small awareness of larger phenomena. Understanding complex music, for example, can be achieved by learning to separately hear its distinct parts. In this case, one experiences a kind of cognitive fine-tuning.

There are limits as to how much you can change—you can't become a musician overnight. You can learn only to do later what you can almost do now. New skills build on existing skills. Growth occurs at the boundaries of your awareness.

Before schools were invented, learning was through apprenticeship and playing in nature. These forms share a multiplicity of scales, time frames, and points of view. In its largest sense, nature contains systems at every scale—many more scales than we're aware of. Nature offers learning situations that cross many boundaries.

The virus is a crash course in environmental education. It has stretched or broken the personality-based structures—like politics and culture—that we build around the idea of control. The virus is the result of a global experiment in production that has made humans vulnerable at many levels. From the virus's point of view, globalism has made humans a resource.

Interconnection

People connect with each other through personality, and modern culture is largely personality-based: it's based on our needs, wants, and vulnerabilities. We've become increasingly less aware of our natural environment as we've become less concerned with it.

We have little control over what we're unaware of, and we're not aware of how vulnerable we've made ourselves to viral transmission and infection. We need to quickly gain more awareness. We need to understand what we've done to enable this virus to appear, infect, and exploit us.

These questions span the gamut ranging from our impact on our environment to how our cells defend themselves. They are not answered by knowing which pharmaceuticals benefit ill patients, which vaccines will protect us, or which policies will restore our economy.

They are not questions being asked by politicians or doctors, although, to give credit where it's due, doctors would like to know all they can in the interest of public health. The same can't be said for politicians struggling for power, using the virus as a weapon.

Science

Science emerged from centuries of conflict between reason and emotion. Science advertised reason over emotion, but there is no such thing. Truth, confidence, certitude, and trust are foundational to science and entirely emotional in nature. Science is an alternative use of emotional reasoning, not a replacement of it (Fleck, 1979).

A battle for hegemony between untrusting allied superpowers has erupted in the virus's theater of war. These same acquisitive efforts infected the cities and the world. Whereas oil is a positive resource for all nations, the virus is a negative resource all nations want to divest from—like a hot potato. It's as if someone pushed the "mutually assured destruction" button and now all nations are fighting for all the spoils left behind.

A vaccine will be developed. It will hold the promise of crowning victorious the nation who possesses it. It will be a messenger RNA based vaccine, similar to other RNA vaccines developed before, none of which have ever been successfully tested or approved (Wood & Spiegle, 2020).

These are genetic modifying agents that rearrange your DNA. They are not medicines. This new accelerated vaccine effort, named "Operation Warp Speed," will skip many of the safety and all of the long-term tests. It will be interesting to see who we're told should take it first (Boodman, 2020).

Ecology

Expand individual engagement through the multiple levels of the ecology.

Things don't end well for a native species when its native ecology changes. And that's what we are and this is what's happening to us. We can either adapt to the new ecology, work to restore the old ecology, or do nothing. Looking for pharmaceutical cures, preventive vaccines, and economic restoratives are the third choice: doing nothing.

Solutions offered by conservationists are a combination of restoring the old ecology while doing nothing about the underlying forces that are upsetting it. Technology, which is mostly reactive and weakly adaptive, does not address the ecological problem.

G5 networks, electric vehicles, advanced weaponry, and other benefits of technology are not ecologically motivated. Adapting to our ecology would mean changing food production and consumption and changing global environmental impact on the land, sea, and air. Few nations can claim any progress on these issues, and globally we can claim none.

The problem is that modern civilization is not designed for environmental sustainability. There have been some civilizations in the past that have done much better, but they had to because they didn't have any alternative. They also didn't have the environmentally destructive potential we have now.

Hypnosis

The remarkable doctor, surgeon, and hypnotherapist, Dabney Ewin, MD, expressed the opinion that almost anything you can treat with cortisone or antihistamine will probably respond to hypnosis (Shenefelt, 2011). Cortisone is a type of steroid. Another steroid drug, dexamethasone, was recently found to reduce deaths by one third for severely ill COVID-19 patients (RECOVERY trial, 2020).

Over a half million people have died worldwide from COVID-19 as of late June 2020. This number continues to rise linearly, as it has for the last three months. I have heard no mention of the use of hypnotherapy for the treatment of COVID-19 at any stage, in spite of its efficacy in emergency medicine (Iserson, 2014). This is my main motivation for writing this book.

The long-term, environmental solution is to change people's awareness. Until people become aware of their ecological danger and grasp how it results from their actions, they won't change their actions.

Many argue for greater understanding, but understanding changes behavior only when it's consistent with desire. Teaching people why they should want what they don't want—even if they understand what you're saying—is a fear-based strategy of questionable merit.

People who love the Earth are already concerned with redressing environmental problems. People who don't have this kind of deep connection with the Earth, or don't want to address the problem, will be motivated to change only when what they do value is threatened.

The hypnosis presented in each of these chapters is a taste of what might be done. These inductions aim to enhance your self-awareness and self-control, and expand your environmental awareness.

Like other forms of learning, hypnosis works by leading you beyond what you already know. You must immerse yourself in it to make new connections between old memories and sensations in order for it to create new feelings and levels of awareness. Once you have experienced these, and their effect has been positive, you won't lose them.

Change

"As above, so below" has become a mystical expression, which is too bad, because it has a long history and a lot of practical meaning. Rejecting "as above, so below" is a rejection of the connection between opposites. This rejection has been a fundamental driving force in Western culture from before Christianity (Kingsley, 1999) and has found its leading proponent in Christianity.

Ecology is the connection of opposites, as well as the connection between many disparate but related elements. The notion of balance is fundamental; and this is not "balance" as in moderation, but balance as in the bringing together of opposites.

It is probably no coincidence that sustainable cultures have been earth-based, or based on earthly deities. That is, they've worshiped nature incarnate rather than a disincarnated divine. It would seem that restoring ecological order calls for a recognition of the ecosystem's importance as both fundamental and, if not sacred, overarching.

Humans have long fought over religion and gotten nowhere, but a conflict between all peoples and the environment—such as this virus and other ecological consequences present—is a conflict of a different order.

The rationalist in me would like to say that developing a sustainable ecology is a practical problem, but I suspect it's not. I suspect it's a spiritual problem, as it certainly is for those who revere the Earth. It requires of people something more than a rational commitment. It is spiritual in the sense that spirit motivates action.

If a microscopic, ubiquitous, almost non-living thing can play a role in altering the minds, values, and behaviors of the Earth's dominant, disruptive species—which is us—then "as above, so below" is more than just a maxim.

> "Religion and philosophy are to be preserved as distinct. We are not to introduce divine revelations into philosophy, nor philosophical opinions into religion."
>
> —**Isaac Newton**, physicist, alchemist, economist, and theologian

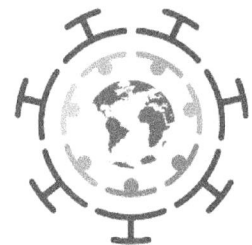

Postscript

This book has four purposes:

First and foremost, the purpose of this book is to introduce hypnosis as a learning and healing tool.

Second, to illustrate and emphasize that, as individuals, we can assert autonomy in how and what we learn, use available information, and reach better conclusions than those offered to us.

Third, to argue that we have reached the limit of our culturally exploitative attitude toward the earth and its resources.

The **forth** and final purpose of this book is to weave these themes into a narrative using my experience with Covid-19.

I hope I have succeeded and that we will take this work further.

Lincoln Stoller, 2020

For more information
follow @LincolnStoller,
#IllnessAndIllumination, and
https://www.mindstrengthbalance.com

THE END

References

Prologue

Humboldt, A. V. (1850) *Views of Nature: or Contemplations on the Sublime Phenomena of Creation*, E. C. Otté and H. G. Bohn trans. London, England: Henry G. Bohn. Retrieved from https://archive.org/details/viewsnatureorco00bohngoog/mode/2up

Szmuda, T., Syed, M. T., Ali, S., Özdemir, C., & Słoniewski, P. (2020, June 15). YouTube as a source of patient information for Coronavirus Disease (COVID −19): A content−quality and audience engagement analysis, *Reviews in Medical Virology. 2020*; e2132. Retrieved from https://doi.org/10.1002/rmv.2132

Chapter 1

Stewart, J. H. (2005). Hypnosis in Contemporary Medicine, *Mayo Clinic Proceedings 80*(4), 511-524.

Chapter 2

Barclay, E., & Scott, D. (2020, March 10). How canceled events and self-quarantines save lives, in one chart, *Vox*. Retrieved from https://www.vox.com/2020/3/10/21171481/coronavirus-us-cases-quarantine-cancellation

Bolin, A. P., Guerra, B. A., Nascimento, S. J. S., & Otton, R. (2012). Changes in lymphocyte oxidant/antioxidant parameters after carbonyl and antioxidant exposure, *International Immunopharmacology*, *14* (4), 690-697. doi:10.1016/j.intimp.2012.10.003. Retrieved from https://www.sciencedirect.com/science/article/pii/S1567576912002950

Briggs, M. (1984). Vitamin C and Infectious Disease: A Review of the Literature and the Results of a Randomized, Double-Blind, Prospective Study Over 8 Years, [1984], in H. M. Briggs (Ed.) *Recent Vitamin Research (1984)* (pp. 39-81). Boca Raton, FL: Taylor and Francis. Retrieved from http://citeseerx.ist.psu.edu/viewdoc/download?doi=10.1.1.444.4873&rep=rep1&type=pdf

DeNoon, D. (2020). The truth about vitamin D: Why you need vitamin D, *WebMD.com*. Retrieved from https://www.webmd.com/osteoporosis/features/the-truth-about-vitamin-d-why-you-need-vitamin-d

Gandhi, M., Yokoe, D.S., & Havlir, D. V. (2020, April 24). Asymptomatic transmission, the Achilles' Heel of current strategies to control Covid-19, *The New England Journal of Medicine, 382,* 2158-2160. Retrieved from https://www.nejm.org/doi/full/10.1056/NEJMe2009758

Harvard School of Public Health (2020, April 1). Ask the expert: The role of diet and nutritional supplements during Covid-19, *Harvard School of Public Health*. Retrieved from https://www.hsph.harvard.edu/nutritionsource/2020/04/01/ask-the-expert-the-role-of-diet-and-nutritional-supplements-during-covid-19/

Koren, E., Kohen, R., & Ginsburg, I. (2010). Polyphenols enhance total oxidant-scavenging capacities of human blood by binding to red blood cells, *Experimental Biology and Medicine (Maywood)*, *235*(6), 689-99. Retrieved from https://www.researchgate.net/publication/44639117_Polyphenols_enhance_total_oxidant-scavenging_capacities_of_human_blood_by_binding_to_red_blood_cells

Lawrence, G. (2020). Breathing, *Gaiam.com*. Retrieved from https://www.gaiam.com/blogs/discover/breathing-is-believing-the-importance-of-nasal-breathing

Levenson, E. (2020, May 19). Staying safe isn't just about hygiene and distance. It's about time, too. *CNN*. Retrieved from https://www.cnn.com/2020/05/18/us/coronavirus-time-risk/index.html

LiveScience, (2020). How does the new coronavirus compare with the flu?, *LiveScience*. Retrieved from https://www.livescience.com/new-coronavirus-compare-with-flu.html

Martineau, A. R., Jolliffe, D. A., Hooper, R. L., Greenberg, Aloia, J. F., Bergman, P., Dubnov-Raz, G., Esposito, S., Ganmaa, D., Ginde, A. A., Goodall, E. C., Grant, C. C., Griffiths, C. J., Janssens, W., Laaksi, I., Manaseki-Holland, S, Mauger, D, Murdoch, D. R., Neale, R., … Camargo, C. A. (2017). Vitamin D supplementation to prevent acute respiratory tract infections: systematic review and meta-analysis of individual participant data, *BMJ, 356*, i6583. doi:10.1136/bmj.i6583. Retrieved from https://www.bmj.com/content/356/bmj.i6583

Martinson, C. (2020). Covid19 – Medicinals, herbals and supplements megathread. *Peak Prosperity Covid19 Library of Files*. Retrieved from https://peakprosperityfilelibrary.wordpress.com/2020/03/13/example-post/

Medical News Today, (2020). How sleep can boost your body's immune response, *Medical News Today*. Retrieved from https://www.medicalnewstoday.com/articles/324432

Pope, T. (2020, March 10). Can I boost my immune system? *New York Times*. Retrieved from http://ww.nytimes.com/2020/03/10/well/live/can-i-boost-my-immune-system.html

Rettner, R. (2020, May 14). How does the new coronavirus compare with the flu? *LiveScience*. Retrieved from https://www.livescience.com/new-coronavirus-compare-with-flu.html

Richardson, S, Hirsch, J., Narasimhan, M., Narasimhan, M.,

Crawford, J. M., McGinn, T., Davidson, K. W., & the Northwell COVID-19 Research Consortium. (2020, April 22). Presenting characteristics, comorbidities, and outcomes among 5700 patients hospitalized with Covid-19 in the New York City area, *JAMA*. doi:10.1001/jama.2020.6775. Retrieved from https://jamanetwork.com/journals/jama/fullarticle/2765184

Science News (2020, May 7). Vitamin D levels appear to play role in Covid-19 mortality rates, *Science News*. Retrieved from https://www.sciencedaily.com/releases/2020/05/200507121353.htm

Walker, M. (2017). *Why We Sleep: The New Science of Sleep and Dreams.* New York, NY: Scribner.

WebMD Medical Reference, (2019). 6 Immune system busters & boosters, *WebMD.com*. Retrieved from https://www.webmd.com/cold-and-flu/cold-guide/10-immune-system-busters-boosters

WHO technical staff (2011, April). Zinc supplementation to improve treatment outcomes among children diagnosed with respiratory infections, *WHO*. Retrieved from https://www.who.int/elena/titles/bbc/zinc_pneumonia_children/en/

Chapter 3

Babo-Rebelo, M., Buot, A., & Tallon-Baudry, C. (2019). Neural responses to heartbeats distinguish self from other during imagination, *NeuroImage*, *191*, 10-20. Retrieved from https://doi.org/10.1016/j.neuroimage.2019.02.012

Besedovsky, L., Lange, T., & Born, J. (2012). Sleep and immune function, *Archiv: European Journal of Physiology, 463*, 121-137. doi:10.1007/s00424-011-1044-0

Lange, T., Bollinger, T., Dimitrov, S., & Diekelmann, S. (2011). Sleep after vaccination boosts immunological memory, *The Journal of Immunology, 187*(1), 283-90. doi:10.4049/jimmunol.1100015

Stoller, L. (2019a). *The Path To Sleep: Exercises for an Ancient Skill.* Victoria, Canada: Mind Strength Balance Press.

Stoller, L. (2019b). *Becoming Lucid: Self-Awareness in Sleeping and Waking Life.* Victoria, Canada: Mind Strength Balance Press.

Chapter 4

Brundage, J. F., & Shanks, G. D. (2008). Deaths from Bacterial Pneumonia during 1918–19 Influenza Pandemic, *Emerging Infectious Diseases, 14*(8),1193-9. doi:10.3201/eid1408.071313

Casanova, L., Alfano-Sobsey, E., Rutala, W. A., Weber, D. J., Sobsey, L., Alfano-Sobsey, E., Rutala, W.A., Weber, D. J., & Sobsey, M. (2008). Virus transfer from personal protective equipment to healthcare employees' skin and clothing, *Emerging Infectious Diseases*, *14*(8), 1291–1293. doi:10.3201/eid1408.080085

Ghose, T. (2020, April 7). How are people being infected with Covid-19? *LiveScience.* Retrieved from https://www.livescience.com/how-covid-19-spreads-transmission-routes.html

Khamsi, R. (2020, March 14). They say coronavirus isn't airborne—But it's definitely borne by air, *Wired Magazine.* Retrieved from https://www.wired.com/story/they-say-coronavirus-isnt-airborne-but-its-definitely-borne-by-air/

Morens, D., Taubenberger, J. K., & Fauci, A. S. (2008). Predominant Role of Bacterial Pneumonia as a Cause of Death in Pandemic Influenza: Implications for Pandemic Influenza Preparedness, *The Journal of Infectious Diseases*, *198* (7), 962–970, https://doi.org/10.1086/591708

Chapter 5

Chapter 6

Brown, R. Q. (2016, August 12). Satisfy your sweet tooth: Natural sugars, *The Whole U, University of Washington*. Retrieved from https://thewholeu.uw.edu/2016/08/12/naturalsugars/

Douard, V., Patel, C., Lee, J., Tharabenjasin, P., Williams, E., Fritton, J. C., Sabbagh, Y., & Ferraris, R. P. (2014, April 9). Chronic high fructose intake reduces serum 1,25 (OH)2D3 levels in calcium-sufficient rodents, *PLOS ONE*. Retrieved from https://doi.org/10.1371/journal.pone.0093611

Mitchell, F. (2020, July). Vitamin-D and Covid-19: Do deficient risk a poorer outcome? *The Lancet Diabetes & Endocrinology 8*(7), 570. Retrieved from https://doi.org/10.1016/S2213-8587(20)30183-2

Chapter 7

Boulware, D. R., Pullen, M. F., Bangdiwala, M. S., Pastick, K. A., Lofgren, S. M., Okafor, E. C., Skipper, C. P., Nascene, A. A., Nicol, M. R., Abassi, N., Engen, N. W., Cheng, M. P., LaBar, D., Lother, S. A., MacKenzie, L. J., Drobot, G., Marten, N., Zarychanski, R., Kelly, L. E., … Hullsiek, K. H. (2020, June 2). A randomized trial of hydroxychloroquine as postexposure prophylaxis for Covid-19, *New England Journal of Medicine*. Retrieved from https://www.nejm.org/doi/full/10.1056/NEJMoa2016638

Citizen's Collective (2020, June 6). Recovery trial: Brexit and overdose, *FranceSoir*. Retrieved from http://www.francesoir.fr/politique-monde/recovery-trial-brexit-and-overdose

Davey, M. (2020, June 12). Covid-19 studies based on flawed Surgisphere data force medical journals to review processes, *The Guardian*. Retrieved from https://www.theguardian.com/world/2020/jun/12/covid-19-studies-based-on-flawed-surgisphere-data-force-medical-journals-to-review-processes

Martinson, C. (2020, April 22). Coronavirus: Debunking the hydroxychloroquine 'controversy' (Dr. Chris Martinson), *Peak Prosperity*. Retrieved from https://www.youtube.com/watch?v=dLSYRqcg0wo

Risch, H. A. (2020, May 27). Early outpatient treatment of symptomatic, high-risk Covid-19 patients that should be ramped-up immediately as key to the pandemic crisis, *American Journal of Epidemiology*. Retrieved from https://academic.oup.com/aje/advance-article/doi/10.1093/aje/kwaa093/5847586

Taggart, A. (2020, May 29). Garbage 'science': Be wary of what you're being told, *Peak Prosperity*. Retrieved from https://www.peakprosperity.com/garbage-science-be-wary-of-what-youre-being-told/

Chapter 8

Gustafson, C., (2017). Bruce Lipton, PhD: The jump from cell culture to consciousness, *Integrated Medicine (Encinitas, Calif.), 16*(6), 44–50. Retrieved from https://www.ncbi.nlm.nih.gov/pmc/articles/PMC6438088/

Hamming, I., Timens, W., Bulthuis, M.L.C., Lely, A. T., Navis, G. J., & van Goor, H. (2004). Tissue distribution of ACE2 protein, the functional receptor for SARS coronavirus. A first step in understanding SARS pathogenesis, *Journal of Pathology. 203*(2), 631-7. doi:10.1002/path.1570

Lawton, G. (2020). Viruses: Viruses are the most abundant organisms on Earth, and probably played a pivotal role in the origin of life, *New Scientist*. Retrieved from https://www.newscientist.com/term/viruses/

Lipton, B. (2018). Crisis ignites evolution. Retrieved from https://www.brucelipton.com/blog/what-world-do-we-live

Rohwer, F., Prangishvili. D., & Lindell, D. (2009). Roles of viruses in the environment, *Environmental Microbiology*, *11*(11), 2771-2774. doi:10.1111/j.1462-2920.2009.02101.x

Wrapp, D., Wang, N., Corbett, K.S., Goldsmith, J. A., Hsieh, C., Abiona, O., Graham, B. S., & McLellan, J. S. (2020). Cryo-EM structure of the 2019-nCoV spike in the prefusion conformation, *Science*, *367*(6483), 1260-1263. doi:10.1126/science.abb2507

Chapter 9

Burdick, A. (2020, June 2). Monster or machine? A profile of the Coronavirus at 6 months, *New York Times*. Retrieved from https://www.nytimes.com/2020/06/02/health/coronavirus-profile-covid.html

Brazil, R. (2014, Sept. 25). The molecules that make memory, *Chemistry World*. Retrieved from https://www.chemistryworld.com/features/the-molecules-that-make-memory/7765.article

Cheek, D. B., & Rossi, E. L. (1994). *Mind-Body Therapy: Methods of Ideodynamic Healing in Hypnosis*. New York, NY: W.W. Norton & Company.

Davis, D. (2007). *The Secret History of the War on Cancer*. New York, NY: Basic Books.

Hudson-Smith, N. (2017, August 18). Royal Rife's universal microscope (and why it can't exist). Retrieved from http://sustainable-nano.com/2017/08/18/royal-rifes-universal-microscope-and-why-it-cant-exist/

Kitman, J. L. (2000, March 2). The secret history of lead, *The Nation*. Retrieved from https://www.thenation.com/article/archive/secret-history-lead/

Reilly, L. (2017, May 17). The most important scientist you've never heard of, *Mental Floss*. Retrieved from https://www.mentalfloss.com/article/94569/clair-patterson-scientist-who-determined-age-earth-and-then-saved-it

Sahl, J., Schönle, A., & Hell, S. W. (2019), Fluorescence microscopy with nanometer resolution. In P. W. Hawkes & J. C. H. Spence (Eds.), *Springer Handbook of Microscopy,* (pp. 1089-1143). Switzerland: Springer Nature.

Schneider, J. M.; Smith, C. W., & Witcher, S. (1984). The relationship of mental imagery to white blood cell (neutrophil) function, *Annual Scientific Meeting of the International Society for Clinical and Experimental Hypnosis*, San Antonio, 1984, pp. 193-216.

Schakel, L., Veldhuijzen, D. S., Crompvoets, P. I., Bosch, J. A., Cohen, S., van Middendorp, H., Joosten, S. A., Ottenhoff, T. H. M., Visser, L. G., & Evers, A. W. M. (2019). Effectiveness of stress-reducing interventions on the response to challenges to the immune system: A meta-analytic review, *Psychotherapy and Psychosomatics, 88*(5), 274–286. doi:10.1159/000501645

Skidel, R. E., & Winter, M. E. (1945). The new microscopes, *Annual Report of the Board of Regents of The Smithsonian Institution-1944*, USGPO. Retrieved from https://www.rife.de/files/smithsonian.pdf

Stoller, L. (2019c). *The Learning Project: Rites of Passage.* Victoria, Canada: Mind Strength Balance Press.

Yamazaki, S., Harata, M., Idehara, T., Konagaya, K., Yokoyama, G., Hoshina, H., & Ogawa, Y. (2020, July 3). Actin polymerization is activated by terahertz irradiation, *Scientific Reports, 8*, 9990. doi:10.1038/s41598-018-28245-9

Vadalà, M., Morales-Medina, J. C., Vallelunga, A., Palmieri, B., Laurino, C., & Iannitti, T. (2016). Mechanisms and therapeutic effectiveness of pulsed electromagnetic field therapy in oncology, *Cancer Medicine 5*(11), 3128–3139. doi:10.1002/cam4.861

Walker, P. (2020). A brief history of the universal microscope. Retrieved from https://www.rife.de/brief_history.html

Zachariae, R., Kristensenb, J. S., Hokland, P., Ellegaard, J., Metze, E., & Hokland, M. (1990). Effect of psychological intervention in the form of relaxation and guided imagery on cellular immune normal healthy subjects, an overview, *Psychotherapy and Psychosomatics 54,* 32-39. Retrieved from https://www.jstor.org/stable/45113773

Chapter 10

Anderson, S. (2020, February). Sex and the microbiome, *Psychology Today.* Retrieved from https://www.psychologytoday.com/ca/blog/mood-microbe/202002/sex-and-the-microbiome

Bongiorno, P. (2014, November). The gut microbiome, anxiety and depression: 6 steps to take, *Psychology Today.* Retrieved from https://www.psychologytoday.com/ca/blog/inner-source/201411/the-gut-microbiome-anxiety-and-depression-6-steps-take

Ferry, B. (2018, January 15). Does Your Gut Hold the Secret to Performance? *Outside.* Retrieved from https://www.outsideonline.com/2274441/no-gut-no-glory

Kinsinger, S. (2017). Cognitive-behavioral therapy for patients with irritable bowel syndrome: Current insights, *Psychology Research and Behavior Management 10*, 231–237. Retrieved from https://www.researchgate.net/publication/318566692_Cognitive-behavioral_therapy_for_patients_with_irritable_bowel_syndrome_Current_insights

Kerry, R., Patra, J. K., Gouda, S., Park, Y., Shin, H., & Das, G. (2018). Benefaction of probiotics for human health: A review, *Journal of Food and Drug Analysis, 26* (3), 927-939. https://doi.org/10.1016/j.jfda.2018.01.002. Retrieved from https://www.sciencedirect.com/science/article/pii/S1021949818300309

Labdoor (2017). Can you overdose on probiotics? Retrieved from https://magazine.labdoor.com/can-you-overdose-on-probiotics

Medicalxpress (2018). Why gut bacteria are essential for a healthy immune system. Retrieved from https://medicalxpress.com/news/2018-03-gut-bacteria-essential-healthy-immune.html

NIH (2020, May 23). Chronic fatigue etiology and recovery in Covid-19 patients: The role of fatigability (FatCovid-19). Retrieved from https://clinicaltrials.gov/ct2/show/NCT04363606

Roman, P., Carrillo-Trabalón, F., Sánchez-Labraca, N., Cañadas, F., Estévez, A. F., & Cardona, D. (2018). Are probiotic treatments useful on fibromyalgia syndrome or chronic fatigue syndrome patients? A systematic review, *Beneficial Microbes*, *9*(4), 603-611. doi:10.3920/BM2017.0125

Shepherd, C. (2020, April 30). Covid-19 and post-viral fatigue syndrome, *ME Association*. Retrieved from https://www.meassociation.org.uk/2020/04/covid-19-and-post-viral-fatigue-syndrome-by-dr-charles-shepherd-30-april-2020/

Venturini, L., Bacchi, S., Capelli, E., Lorusso, L., Ricevuti, G., & Cusa, C. (2019). Modification of Immunological parameters, oxidative stress markers, mood symptoms, and well-being status in CFS patients after probiotic intake: Observations from a pilot study, *Oxidative Medicine and Cellular Longevity*, *2019*. Retrieved from https://doi.org/10.1155/2019/1684198

Wolf, C. (2016, January 7). Did probiotics cure my chronic fatigue syndrome? *Health Rising*. Retrieved from https://www.healthrising.org/blog/2016/01/07/probiotics-cure-my-chronic-fatigue-syndrome/

Yong, E. (2020, June 4). COVID-19 can last for several months, *The Atlantic*. Retrieved from https://www.theatlantic.com/health/archive/2020/06/covid-19-coronavirus-longterm-symptoms-months/612679/

Chapter 11

Griffith, D. (2020, March 23). We are the meaning makers. Retrieved from https://lorian.org/community/2020/3/21/we-are-the-meaning-makers

Humboldt, A. (1846). *Cosmos: Sketch of a Physical Description of the Universe, Vol. I*, London, England: Longman, Brown, Green and Longmans.

Sagan, C., Malone, A., Druyan, A., Soter, Steven, Gibson, Kent (Eds.) (1980). *Cosmos by Carl Sagan: a Personal Voyage.*

Chapter 12

Walls, L. D., Jackson, S. T., & Person, M. W. (2014). Introduction: Reclaiming consilience. *Views of Nature, Alexander von Humboldt.* Chicago, IL: U. of Chicago Press.

Chapter 13

Boodman, E. (2020, March 11). Researchers rush to test coronavirus vaccine in people without knowing how well it works in animals, *STAT Health.* Retrieved from https://www.statnews.com/2020/03/11/researchers-rush-to-start-moderna-coronavirus-vaccine-trial-without-usual-animal-testing/

Fleck, R. (1979). *The Genesis and Development of a Scientific Fact.* Chicago, IL: U. of Chicago Press.

Iserson, K. V. (2014). An hypnotic suggestion: Review of hypnosis for clinical emergency care, *Journal of Emergency Medicine*, *46*(4). doi:10.1016/j.jemermed.2013.09.024. Retrieved from https://www.researchgate.net/publication/259959216_An_Hypnotic_Suggestion_Review_of_Hypnosis_for_Clinical_Emergency_Care

Kingsley, P. (1999). *In the Dark Places of Wisdom.* Point Reyes Station,

CA: Golden Sufi Center Publishing.

RECOVERY trial (2020, June 16). Low-cost dexamethasone reduces death by up to one third in hospitalized patients with severe respiratory complications of Covid-19. Retrieved from https://www.recoverytrial.net/files/recovery_dexamethasone_statement_160620_v2final.pdf

Shenefelt, P. D. (2011). Ideomotor signaling: From divining spiritual messages to discerning subconscious answers during hypnosis and hypnoanalysis, a historical perspective, *American Journal of Clinical Hypnosis*, *53*(3), 157-167.

Thomas, M. (2018, March 15). To control your life, control what you pay attention to, *Harvard Business Review*. Retrieved from https://hbr.org/2018/03/to-control-your-life-control-what-you-pay-attention-to

Wood, G., & Spiegle, D. A. (2020, March 21). Covid-19 vaccines are coming, but they're not what you think, *The Atlantic*. Retrieved from https://www.theatlantic.com/ideas/archive/2020/03/two-extreme-long-shots-could-save-us-coronavirus/608539/

About the Author

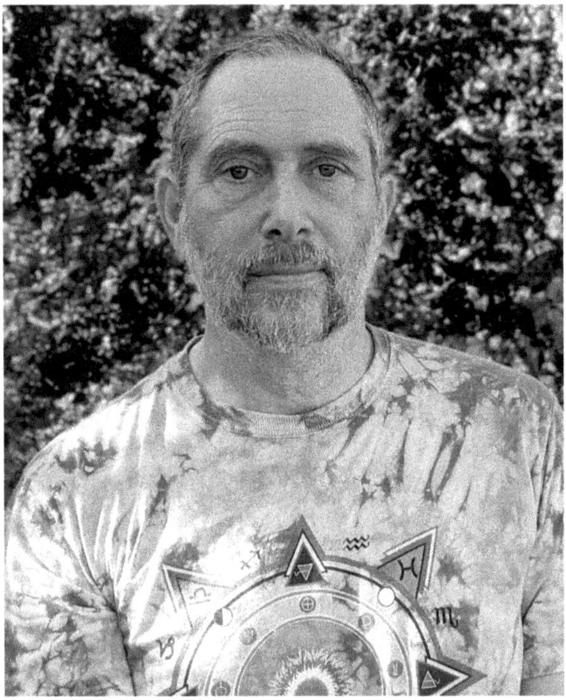

Lincoln Stoller has published work as a physicist, astronomer, statistician, biologist, neurophysiologist, neurofeedback therapist, psychologist, hypnotherapist, computer scientist, software architect, anthropologist, mountaineer, and educator. He has built two houses and has licenses to pilot soarplanes, fly paragliders, and scuba dive.

He holds a PhD in quantum physics from the University of Texas, hypnotherapy certifications from ICBCH and IMDHA, and the patent for the design of a business accounting system which he programmed and supported for 15 years. He is an assessing editor at the Journal of Mind and Behavior.

Lincoln has spent 40 years involved with various schools of spirituality and mediation, 20 years with the therapeutic and religious use of psychedelics, 10 years offering EEG brainwave training, and the last 5 years as a hypnotherapist in private practice specializing in medical support, sleep enhancement, spiritual guidance, and business psychology. All of which is to say, he helps people learn things. His previous three books are: *The Learning Project, Rites of Passage*; *The Path To Sleep*; and *Becoming Lucid*.

His 22-year-old son Kiran lives with Lincoln's ex-wife in New York, and his 10-year-old son Pythagoras lives with Lincoln in Victoria, British Columbia, Canada, to which he moved for educational and political reasons, and to be closer to mountains, forests, and the sea.

www.ingramcontent.com/pod-product-compliance
Lightning Source LLC
Chambersburg PA
CBHW051540020426
42333CB00016B/2027
9781999253851